Bipolar 1 Disorder

How to Survive and Thrive

Molly McHugh

www.mollymchugh.com

Dedication

For all those who have suffered with mental health issues, especially bipolar illness, and all who have written about and shared their experiences.

I hope this sharing helps you or a loved one as much as reading those memoirs helped me on many occasions.

Disclaimer

This book is a memoir. I am sharing my personal story and the information contained within this book is true and factual to the best of my memory. It contains snapshots of my life with a focus on my experiences living with the illness Bipolar 1 Disorder. It's not a pretty picture much of the time and was not an easy story to tell.

Humor is one of my better personality traits and I tried to weave some amusement in with the tragic events I have lived through. I do not consider my life as a whole tragic but mental illness has made living life very difficult at times.

I also share alternative medical treatments I have done to treat the bipolar as well as a form of CFS/ME I live with. This book is not intended to be medical advice. I am not a licensed health care provider. I am simply one of an approximate 5.5 million Americans 18 or older who have been diagnosed bipolar.

We all have our unique stories to tell, this is mine.

Table of contents

CHAPTER 1
How it all Started 8

CHAPTER 2
What Bipolar Illness is Really Like 16

CHAPTER 3
Diagnosis Manic Depression 24

CHAPTER 4
Is it OK to Discriminate Against Someone Diagnosed
Bipolar? 32

CHAPTER 5
Mania & Hypomania 52

CHAPTER 6
Hospitalizations & Getting Better 63

CHAPTER 7
Playing Doctor Roulette 71

CHAPTER 8
The Lithium Cure That Didn't Work 78

CHAPTER 9
Bipolar Disorder vs Drug Addiction 87

CHAPTER 10
Relapse, Suicide Risk & Times Past 97

CHAPTER 11
Bipolar Onset, Acknowledging Illness & Contributing Factors
.... 110

CHAPTER 12
Is Bipolar I Disorder More Severe Than Bipolar II Disorder?
.... 119

CHAPTER 13
Major Depression is Hell 129

CHAPTER 14
Things That Helped Me That May Help You or a Loved One
.... 140

CHAPTER 15
Treatments & Self Help Protocols 149

CHAPTER 16
Learning to Separate Yourself From Illness.........................176

CHAPTER 17
Social Life & Relationships...180

CHAPTER 18
Care, Concern & Love..188

CHAPTER 19
We Will Skip the Torture 195

CHAPTER 20
Living Life & Moving On 204

CHAPTER 1

How it all Started

It was a cloudy day in San Francisco, maybe rainy maybe not. Feeling a little down, more work ahead for the afternoon and evening I headed back to the dorms after class. I rode the elevator to Phelan Hall #4 and stepped off.

There he was. My beloved teddy bear, hanging limply from the ceiling right in front of me, swaying back and forth slowly. His fuzzy, light brown head was tilted off to the side, hanging down past his shoulders, looking looser than a stuffed animal's head should; white, terry cloth bathrobe belt noose strung around his neck and all.

I had to laugh and plans for revenge began. Nothing new, but this prank by fun-loving friends would turn into an unknowing omen of what I would feel like doing to myself on occasion for the rest of my life. And it wasn't so funny. Weeks later I would experience my first episode of Bipolar I Disorder. And these same friends would end up calling every psychiatric ward within city limits searching for me so they could visit.

That's how it all started. At least before I knew what

depression was and that weeks before I snapped into a psychosis I was experiencing the start of one. Not really a snap, but more like a very quick progression. Not having much experience with altered states of mind of any sorts, I was clueless to the signs of an impending manic psychosis. Nineteen years old, away in a new city, new college. As is the norm, first time living away from home, on my own.

And at a school I never visited prior to attending or researched thoroughly. Led merrily through a Catholic upbringing with 12 years at private Catholic schools under my belt, it's no wonder I ended up at a private, Jesuit university. And with my experiences at this school, it is no wonder I was led away from this faith, never to return again.

It started out innocently enough. It was a bright, sunny spring. I was living on the university's small, inner city, tree-filled campus, enjoying life, beginning to prepare for final exams which were a few weeks away. First time living out of Washington State, the new varieties of allergens and pollens hit me hard. I was popping antihistamines on schedule four times or more daily depending on how much I had to study.

If I didn't my eyes would water and itch so much I couldn't read a thing, much less actually concentrate and process information. Whatever someone had on hand I would take. I knew how important exercise was and kept up going for runs in and around Golden Gate Park and swimming at the local pool even though I didn't feel all that great.

Motivated to do well regardless of not feeling great, I thought more time studying was the answer. Diligence wasn't getting the results I needed so I went in with a friend on purchase of some speed then pulled an all-nighter to cram two months of undigested physiology material into my under functioning brain for an exam the next day. We both aced it.

Much better results yet not very long-lasting. Even though I took very little drug, and for only one night it was enough to help push me on my way towards what I would learn to be my unknown genetic inheritance: Manic Depressive illness.

A few days before the last set of tests of the year I wound-up beyond return. I was taking what I thought at the time were BRILLIANT photos. Not just good snap shots but mind-boggling visions of objects; abstract, with the perfect shade of light. Objects around my room, scenes of downtown San Francisco mirrored in the wall length window, bathed in early evening light.

I dorm hopped a few parties feeling higher than high (but not on any illegal substances) shooting rolls of film of partying friends. I was abnormally anxious and hyper, not drinking much. And anyways, who needed alcohol? I had important things to complete i.e. the cool photos I was taking of all the cool people I knew. And they were dazzling, exceptional shots. I could not WAIT to see the processed film I would get to see a few days later.

I didn't feel like partying but couldn't stop moving and doing. Regardless of my internal state I fit in very well, smiles all around. That's the last sane—if you can call it that—thing I really remember.

Things started to go weird. A lunch in the cafeteria turned into a hallucinogenic trip back to the dorm. I wasn't hungry, feeling nauseous mainly, but tried to make myself eat regardless. I wasn't really ill in the normal physical sense—no known flu or fever—but my body was undergoing a biochemical change that was making me feel sick.

My brain was malfunctioning. I didn't hear voices or see visions yet was in an altered state beyond my control. Hysterically laughing one minute about something that may have amused me a little before then confused and placid the next, with no clue as to what was transpiring in-between or in total.

Uncontrollable laughter and mood swings known only to those who can reach the highs of mania. I walked out of a final exam fully out of it. I was unable to think of even lame, passable answers to the few test questions I read. I don't remember who finally clued in or why, but not long after I was led to the counseling center terrified beyond belief; I had no idea what was happening to me.

Flying high I was projecting my fears and issues at warp speed to anything and everything around me... imagining a few as well. Things that most 19 year olds get to work through at a bit slower pace, over the course of a few years, not in an hour.

First, I had some strange premonition that I was getting married. And that was terrifying (as it should have been, I didn't even have a steady guy at the time). A good, conservative (yet neurotic) Catholic mother made sure to tell me at least once a month during my teen years how 'sex was for marriage'. I was playing around a bit, had a couple intense crushes and somehow the possibility of accomplishing the full act brought up a tad bit of anxiety during my over-processing episode.

Then the counselor looked creepy to me and I felt uncomfortable (that was a bit sane considering the situation). Why was I taken to this dungeon office (lower level of building next door) that I had never been in before? Who is this man asking me questions that I could barely hear or mentally process much less answer? I looked at him and was sure he was gay and that somehow was a major, terrifying issue, and I was so extra-perceptive to see it, had to blurt it out.

I couldn't help but blurt out my brilliant insights as they flashed through my brain. Yet nothing really fazed me for long; one mental event zipped to the next at light speed before I could even really process either. And I knew EVERYTHING and was so smart. And it was a very scary feeling. I don't think I cried, don't think I could have, but maybe did. Every ounce of my being was in hyper alert, and for what reason I had no idea. I was trapped inside a mind-body connection the likes of which I'd never experienced or witnessed before.

Then the fun really started. Taken by car to a crisis center, I was asked a few questions and given a major tranquilizer. Not long after, I started to stabilize. I was crashing down slowly but enough to realize that during the hours (and days) before I had been experiencing something different and now was starting to feel normal again.

The craziness was subsiding and my old self was re-surfacing. I told a nurse "I am fine now" and remember all too well the laugh that was her reply. At the time her battle-hardened attitude was crushing to my very naive and new state of confusion; I couldn't understand why I wasn't being listened to, much less laughed at.

I'd always been a fairly sane (though crazy fun at times like most teenagers) and responsible person with few major problems living in the world up until that time... what was different now? How had things changed? I was shoved into a whole new category of existence against my will—that of a mental patient.

I was put in a wheelchair, given another dose of downers regardless of my wishes and vocalized opposition and put into the back of a van; strapped in like a quadriplegic and driven across the bay to a mental hospital outside of the city.

The van was fully equipped with a security, metal mesh screen divider between the back area containing me and the back and front passenger seats like they were transporting high-risk jail cargo instead of a sick, helpless and very scared person. And for what? I was going to chew the thick leather straps off with my teeth, pull a blow torch out of my back pocket, melt a hole through the divider and go and... laugh the driver to death?

Or more likely, collapse on the back seat in a fit of antipsychotic drug-induced stupor? Who knows. The only important thing at the time for all those in charge of my well-being seemed to be that where we were going they could keep me overnight. Lucky me.

CHAPTER 2

What Bipolar Illness
is Really Like

Experiencing bipolar illness is like being hit by a freight train when you knowingly didn't step on any tracks—over and over again. You lose your self—your normal, functioning self—for periods of time regardless of what you do, didn't do, or have done. At least that is what it is like for me.

Getting hit by states of mind that are beyond your control and for what reason you have no idea. Numbing depression with unrelenting fatigue that turns a 24 hour period into a haze of wakefulness and lethargy. You remain lethargic regardless of what needs to be done, the importance of what needs to be done or your desire to get things done.

A depressive state that can last for days, weeks or months. You never know when it will end. You do not know when your brain will revert back into that 'normal, functioning self' mode. Or whether a switch is on the way and things will cycle out of control.

Worse, in my opinion, is getting back to normal then speeding up. Your thoughts start moving quicker and it seems normal to you inside your head but talking to people starts to get a little off. Your speech is too quick. You interrupt the other person talking when not intending to though you do or don't really care, depending on how wound up you happen to be.

More importantly your power is coming back. You're waking up again. It feels good, but may be embarrassing at times. No bother. You know it's a little 'off' for you, but move through that quickly as well; too quickly, no time to be self-conscious. The other person, if there is an other person, rarely has a clue to what is going on. Nothing crazy going on here, at least not yet.

You start not wanting to communicate (to others, so as not to embarrass yourself). Or you get aggressive and hot-headed, trying to maintain this state of mind which seems so enjoyable. Now the effort is on focus and concentration, to hold it together while enjoying immensely what's going on in your head. Now I can think!

And it's brilliant. You are not depressed and worthless, you're high-functioning and moving forward. All those things to get done and do. The groundbreaking ideas and start of long, thought about projects are on their way. Where did I put that list? What should I be working on again?

During one such time it was my brilliant book complete with brilliant title "Diary of a Psych Patient" (which at times was also very, very funny). Other times it has been my brilliant ideas on what is wrong with the world and how to fix it. Or at least I get to the 'what is wrong' part and catch up with recent world events. I just need to concentrate, work, focus…

Then I will get something accomplished, get to feel a sense of accomplishment other than simply surviving a down time. Sometimes this happens but most often not.

Not at least in my case when this rapid cycling was occurring and I did not have the words or understanding to identify what it was. I knew what rapid cycling was and that I was not one of those types of bipolar patients. Or was I? I may have not presented that way clinically but it was a lot of what was going on internally, and why I was suicidal during my 20s off and on. I also had a chronic pain syndrome that was exacerbating the depressive episodes.

It seemed it was never going to end. And it didn't until I could find aids to help stabilize my brain chemistry. At this time the mood states were on the extreme end of the bipolar illness spectrum and fluctuations between states happened often. Avoiding being hospitalized was a primary concern, accomplishing goals came in a distant yet hopeful second.

When the hypomanic phase is at its hilt, especially when it is a rebound phase after a serious depressive episode, I was usually more erratic than highly functional. I was not necessarily dysfunctional to an outside observer and could get the basic tasks of day to day living completed with some pleasure and enjoyment but my internal state was not stable.

Not stable in that I'm still jumping off the inner walls of my psyche, bouncing around a bit, trying to process the new chemical structure which is defining my existence at that time. The chemical structure that is not defining my self, but that is setting the parameters that self gets to muddle around in.

This was especially true during my early 20s when the illness was taking the heaviest toll on my life. A heavy toll on my developing psyche, self and life as a young adult growing up in the United States. Until I found things that helped me stabilize, helped lessen the extreme mood states and gave periods of stability long enough to get a foothold on something in life. Time to accomplish a goal or two, make new friends, move forward in life. Before that time I was a bit of a psychological mess.

Ok, I'll give a little... at times I am now (writing this book in 2015) too.

In the hypomanic states I would spend days with the mind racing going on, loving the feel good time I was having—with myself or others. Loving the ability to think, to process thought; my brilliant thoughts. Not going to give this up. Forget it. Time with others is more fun. You laugh, make jokes, feel like you 'have your brain back'.

During these times the brain may feel like it is back, kicked into gear again but that normal, functioning self is being a bit overridden. She's in there somewhere, not that I really care at this point. I care, but it is easier to say I don't because it is emotionally painful. Too frustrating to be stuck in this mental rut and not be able to get myself out. Pull myself up by those bootstraps and get on with my life. "How pathetic am I?" the self asks.

If I think of things to be done, I get so many items on my list that I get overwhelmed. The list running in my brain. At this point I am not organized or calm enough to write things down and slowing down really isn't an option. Or I am too fatigued to write. And just happy that I don't feel as bad as I did the days, weeks before.

Most often I'm ecstatic with being able to think, period. Connect with the real world, that'll come. I want to enjoy the time I am having not in the depressive state anymore which was hell and get the most out of it. Things will get done, everything is going to be fine. I can handle this.

Those hypomanic states soothe the rough edges of the prior depression, heal the soul a bit. You start to actually care about things and participate in life. You aren't thinking of leaving the planet anymore, researching what drug cocktail would accomplish that goal or how and where to buy a gun.

As your mood lifts from that dark hole a beacon of your self shines through. Your normal functioning self is back and you have hope. The future looks bright.

Often at this time a desire for retrospection sets in, albeit often overdone. It goes something like this: "Now I can actually figure out what the heck my problem is, why I get depressed, all the solutions to those problems, and for everyone else who experiences these problems... and will never be ill again."

The hypomania and all its associated thoughts and feelings hasn't had time to fully emit, to level out. The train is back on the tracks but still going a little over the speed limit; 40 miles per hour in a 30 mile per hour zone. And it feels good. I'm on top of the heap, back in the saddle and what do I want out of life anyways, now that I actually feel like living it to some extent. Things don't seem so bad.

I feel good as I'm connected to life again. I enjoy interacting with others, enjoy the sights, sounds and smells penetrating my senses that I was oblivious to before. That tastes good. I've always wanted to learn how to make Pad Thai. I haven't gone for a run in a while. I really need to start exercising again. I don't mind a little rain. The raindrops are beautiful reflecting off the light hitting the rearview mirror of that parked car.

I am not pushed into a black, separate hole outside of the mainstream. I am a part of life, a part of the otherness of this world and have value. I'm not just stuck in my own mind, feeling awful; not anymore.

Time moves forward and as long as a relapse is kept at bay so does my life. I get philosophical about financial losses, feel appreciative of the high functioning times I've been fortunate to have. I am thankful I finally finished that college degree and for the challenging, well-paid work it led to. Thankful for the ruggedly handsome, fun to party with but didn't talk a whole lot Norwegian fisherman who got me knocked up (other thoughts about this on other occasions) and giving birth to a beautiful, healthy baby boy.

So what if that's not what is really deemed as success by society when the job losses, lack of a significant other (wasn't I supposed to be married by now?), lack of much social life (why am I still so tired all the time?), brief psychiatric hospitalizations, months on welfare assistance and periods of homelessness get calculated in.

I feel good, things are looking up.

CHAPTER 3

Diagnosis Manic Depression

I walked the same way home I always did after my weekend shift as a waitress at a local Haight-Ashbury Café; nonchalantly, glad the shift was over. After a few moments enjoying the fresh air and colorful townhouses I loved to look at and envision myself living in one day I turned a corner and started the four blocks left to traverse before reaching my shared apartment.

As I did I felt compelled to look up and then down the street. I noticed someone standing outside on the sidewalk a couple of blocks ahead.

I kept walking as usual and they kept standing there, not moving. One more extended block later I was walking past the person, whom I could now identify as a 30 year or so old woman. The person turned to me and said, with a slight smile on her face, "There's a fire." That was it. Looked at me, spoke those words then turned and casually walked up the stairs and into the house.

I was very confused. If there was a fire why was the woman smiling? Something was incredibly wrong with this picture. The woman had stood around for five to seven minutes waiting for me to approach and was not acting alarmed in any way whatsoever but obviously wanted me to follow her into the house.

I stood on the sidewalk for a few minutes longer, not sure what was happening or what I should do. I looked up at the house and saw a tuft of smoke coming out of a window after she had entered, but no sign of any flames, no persons calling out in distress. It's a setup, my sixth sense told me, and I walked away down the street to my apartment feeling more than a little disturbed.

My main conclusion at that point was that the woman was mentally disturbed, on some type of drug, or both. Forty minutes or so later I heard sirens. Someone had called the fire department. That did wonders for my fear/guilt that was now escalating. What if I had left someone in distress that needed help?

I walked the two blocks back to the corner and looked up the street where the house was. No signs of any burning building, just a few firemen standing around. I turned and walked away, feeling a bit better but not for long. 'I'm truly insane', passed through my mind as well as 'what was that'?

What had happened was bizarre but if it was an actual setup, what would have happened to me if I had gone into the house? Gang raped, murdered? I didn't have an enemy to speak of, why would someone want to cause me harm?

Conveniently, and as luck would have it, I had an ear to vent my initial fear turned post incident hysteria on: my Abnormal Psychology class professor who I knew used to be a cop. I had to tell someone.

I visited his office one afternoon shortly after the incident and recounted the basics of what happened, overwhelmed with emotion and anxiety. That wasn't too out of the norm for me at the time. I was (still am) a highly sensitive person and prone to nervousness when the comfort zone of myself is pushed out of her comfort zone. It is possible 'hysterics' was the primary thought that crossed his mind but that is not for me to say or know.

He did not instruct me to make a report to the police, or anything of that sort, seemed more concerned about my state of mind and the level of anxiety I was expressing than events that had transpired. The short talk did little to alleviate my concerns.

Next stop the office of Dr. S—the psychiatrist who had seen me one and a half years previously in the throes of my psychotic break. On the bus to a transfer station downtown, ticket purchase in hand and onto the Transbay Tube underwater rail system I went. Across the bay connecting the city of San Francisco to Oakland, back to the same inpatient facility I had spent a fitful night in.

It was where Dr. S had his office. I wasn't thrilled about having to make the appointment (my decision alone, no one made me or even suggested it) but at least this time I wasn't strapped into a wheelchair when entering through the front doors.

I was questioning my sanity and he did a bit as well. He listened to my recount of the experience and to symptoms I had been experiencing such as fatigue, excessive daytime drowsiness where I got sleepy to the point of wanting to pass out. He came to the conclusion that I was in the depressive phase of a full-blown Category 1 Manic Depressive Illness. He'd already seen me in the manic/psychotic stage.

Now the diagnosis was official. I was told I was Manic Depressive after the spring of Freshman Year hospitalization but knew that the official title on the books was 'atypical psychosis'. It could have been indicative as a first stage of many forms of illness. It takes time to assess true bipolar illness and give an accurate diagnosis though the illness itself has been around for ages.

The below is quoted from *BPhope.com: Through the Ages, It's Been There*.

"Measurable progress was made in the early 1850s when Jean-Pierre Falret, a French psychiatrist, identified folie circulaire or circular insanity—manic and melancholic episodes that were separated by symptom-free intervals. He broke substantial new academic ground when he chronicled distinct differences between simple depression and heightened moods. In 1875, because of his work, the term "manic-depressive psychosis," a psychiatric disorder, was coined. Scientists also credit Falret with recognizing a genetic link associated with this disease."

Source: BPhope.com

http://www.bphope.com/Item.aspx/162/through-the-ages-its-been-there

I was a good patient, accepted the diagnosis and already knew the protocol for treatment as a nursing student. Even though I understood I was diagnosed with a mood disorder, I often questioned what was going on with me. What bothered me most was the daytime drowsiness that improved off and on but was significantly affecting my life. I was tired often, though looked well from the outside.

At age 20 you do not want to be about to pass out at three in the afternoon (no alcohol involved, I hardly drank then except when out with friends), drag through the rest of the day trying to get work done and enjoy life a bit, then exhausted by 8 p.m.

The summer ended and back to school I went, now in my third year of the four year baccalaureate program. First up was a clinical rotation in Psychiatry. The previous year I had clinical rotations in Pediatrics and in Obstetrics/Gynecology. Both went well. The OB/GYN instructor was not only highly skilled and experienced with years spent teaching at the university, but also one of the nicest, kindest ladies you would want to meet.

She had all of her students over to her home one day, and I remember her showing us how she nursed her children when they were infants. On the couch, baby against the back of the couch, her on her side facing baby, pillows arranged just so. That way, regardless of how exhausted she may have been, if she fell asleep she would not have rolled onto (and suffocated) her child; very smart.

Even though we were 'just nursing students' it was a very heady experience to be in the hospital working as a temporary staff member. The real staff just kept out of the way for the most part, glad I am sure to have many of the basic tasks of

29

caring for the patients handled by these newbies and their workload reduced. We rarely saw or communicated with doctors but when that did happen was even more of a high.

During the Pediatrics rotation I was assigned one day to care for a baby girl of one of the physicians who worked at the Veterans Affairs (VA) hospital in the city. Talk about nervous. She was in for observation and tests as cried and cried and they could not figure out what—if anything—was wrong. The poor guy, and I am sure his wife, was exhausted from driving around the city trying to get her to sleep.

One morning on the elevator we rode in it together, exchanged hellos. Ok, this isn't such a big deal I thought, no need to be nervous. It is just work training and I am clearly doing a good job if I'm getting these assignments.

Now in year three of the program, Psychiatry and General Medicine clinical rotations were next up to bat. Upon completion of the year I would have been eligible to take the state licensing exams for the State of California. The fourth year was more theory, some advanced training and for many ambitious students preparation to continue on to graduate school.

CHAPTER 4

Is it OK to Discriminate Against Someone Diagnosed Bipolar?

For the first time we were actually asked what we wanted to do during the semester. The first year of clinical (second year in the program) you were just assigned an instructor, told where to meet and when to start the rotation. And that was that. Up at 5:30 a.m., to the cafeteria for a quick bite to eat and then meet-up with whoever had a car.

I said I wanted to work with children. It seemed like the best fit since it was what I had some experience in. I had no experience with mental illness at that point other than my own and was doing ok. I thought working with kids would be less stressful, less of a trigger to what I had experienced years earlier.

Instead I was assigned to a lockdown, crisis facility psych ward at the UCSF Medical Center for adults. They housed the sickest of the sick. For most of this population the revolving door syndrome would end in placement in a long term psychiatric institution, life on the streets or an early death. Administering high doses of psychiatric meds was the main name of the game.

The night before the first day my inner self was expressing a little apprehension. 'I have a mental illness, one false step and they will put me away, lock the door and throw away the key'. 'No, they won't'. 'You are fine, everything will be fine.'

Sitting at my desk around 11 p.m. after staying up late to finish a paper due the following afternoon I knew I should have gone to bed but didn't. Instead I pushed the greasy popcorn bowl off to the side, drained my coffee cup for the fourth or fifth time and tried to think of any idioms I could come up with. Knowing that was one diagnostic tool used at the time to separate the sane from insane I was trying to insure I would get to leave the ward at the end of that first day.

'A bird in hand is worth two in the bush'. Got it. 'A leopard can't change his spots'. No problem. 'Actions speak louder than words'. Mentally exhausted, a couple of the phrases threw me for a loop which of course only increased my anxiety level. 'Oh god, they are definitely going to put me away'.

My concerns were unwarranted and when the steel-reinforced door slammed shut and locked behind me at the end of the day, I was grateful to know that I was leaving and heading back to my apartment. The apartment just three blocks from Golden Gate Park that I shared with a fun gal who was a science wiz, did well in school and was almost always smiling and cheerful (unlike me).

She took our spaghetti sauce making competitions as seriously as I did; both adamantly claiming victory every time. The secret is to add some ground sausage, not just hamburger... and some fresh, chopped tomatoes, not just canned.

I was also grateful that when I had experienced a breakdown I wasn't brought there. Sometimes when life has dealt a crushing blow it is comforting to have the awareness that things could be, or could have been, worse.

The instructor I was assigned to was new at the university and we were her first class of students. Up until this time all the instructors in the program were nice, professional and had worked at the school for years. This gal was a bit different. She wasn't sincerely nice but plenty phony nice. Phony at least to me; other students whom came from wealthy families she drooled over with attention. I've nicknamed her The Drone.

The Drone pretended to be nice when in the presence of others. When I had to be alone with her she was cold and aloof, almost hostile. It was as if I was an object, a thing, something she had to interact with but for some reason did not want to. Was it because she had been told I had experienced a mental breakdown?

She never showed any real concern or care for the mental health patients on the ward. Not at the inpatient facility, not at the childcare center for teen mothers I had to work at or for the individual couple who were living with mental health issues independently that I was assigned to go visit.

She was just a PhD drone i.e. someone who had worked hard, was ambitious but lacked real intelligence and now was set upon society in the role she had trained for.

The Drone ignored me for the most part and I did not like her much though knew I really didn't have to. I only had to do what I was asked to do as a student and be professional. She was phony and the staff at the ward didn't seem to like her much either.

It was simple work and the weeks went by quickly. The patients were low income or homeless and most had been ill for years. As nursing students we observed, sat in on the meetings with the attending psychiatrist and administered meds to the patients we were assigned to care for. I think we handed out meds during this rotation. In clinical settings there were things nursing students could and could not do. Give meds and shots, yes. Start an IV? No.

One of these patients was transferred to a long-term facility that as part of the curricula we visited one day. As we walked through the dismal ward with its dirty-white walls and large, vacant room with a glaring lack of furniture I recognized him. We were all standing around in a circle listening to droneville and he was standing off to the side alone, looking over at the group with no one acknowledging his presence.

The Drone was intentionally ignoring him and the scene going on did not feel right to me, like I was participating in something I did not want to participate in.

'Just because this person has a mental illness that has not been treated successfully and he cannot function in society does not mean he has no value or worth as a human being;

that he deserves to be mistreated'—was my line of thought at the time.

I addressed him when there was a lull in the conversation and said hello, asked how he was. I thought that was appropriate since we were going to be nurses and supposed to actually care about these people and their welfare. The Drone shot me a look of disgusted hostility. I was confused, what did I do wrong? Nothing. The Drone was simply acting out her hostility towards me, not my action; or quite possibly both.

Meanwhile, back at the ranch—my life outside the nursing program—things were ok but not great. I wasn't necessarily unhappy but was bored with coursework that was very time consuming yet uninteresting and I was lonely. Why wasn't I meeting anyone, dating much? This 'going out with friends and trying to' routine was becoming a drag.

My love life was definitely a drag. Drag, disappointment, let down… and it was not like I didn't put in a little effort into the romance department. Let's do a quick recap. I'll reminisce while you get to sit back and read.

First there was visiting a high school friend who got early admittance to Santa Clara University in California. My first time on an airplane (wow, what a high that was) when I went for a weekend visit. Outdoor swimming pool on campus, lots of toned bodies and falling off a barstool at a dark, dingy local pub. More like slipped off to the side, drunk and lip-locked with a college hottie whom I never wanted to part from.

He couldn't be a keeper. I was on a plane back to Seattle the next day. But I sure was looking forward to this thing called college.

Then freshman orientation at POS.U. Local guy (not a hottie, but passable) working the parties to find some innocent newbie to hit on and found me. Took me out—I had a date!—riding around the city on his motorcycle and to dinner. More high (he drove fast) then back to the dorms and lots of heavy petting with a few personal boundaries now a thing in the past. College was fun!

Then a night with a bunch of wealthy Europeans and however sophisticated I thought I may be or tried to be, did not fit in. Out of my league is a phrase that fits. But this species of male was more than I'd been accustomed to. The boyfriend I'd been with back home and thinking he'd be a great catch now paled in comparison. He was sweet and I was attached but not ready for any type of commitment and these guys made my insides turn in ways they hadn't been turned.

My confidence improved some and I landed one; an adorable German guy named Moritz. Fun, full of energy, easy to be around—he's my type, I thought. We walked hand in hand down the Haight Ashbury one day. Kissed on the sidewalk while the rest of the world passed by. Made me feel like all was right in the world.

I wanted him to be the one. He wanted my crimson red colored, faded pants (not joking, they were really cool jeans and he was really artsy) more than he wanted me and to be in mine. Friend status never progressed beyond just that. He found a super hot art student to hang out with and moved on. I was a bit crushed.

But if college is good for one thing, it's all kinds of opportunity. Landed another hottie (for a few hours this time, not just two) who was older and on the baseball team. I must be special. Making-out on the street outside the bar, another high. College is the jam.

We walked back to the dorms. He wants to come inside. I can't. Get busy with roommate in bed 12 feet away? That's weird. And how busy was I supposed to be getting? I'm in over my head with this one.

Next year forced to live on POS.U campus though wanted to move into a house a few blocks away with a friend. Low rent, my own room plus a kitchen equals score! Fascist POS.U (this was the 80s) decided women and men needed to be segregated. College sophomores were not mature enough to share a hallway with members of the opposite sex, it seems. Or to live off-campus. My request was denied.

Yet POS.U thought us very capable of being forced to pay their exorbitant housing costs and take out costly Federal subsidized loans. Side note: the dorm cafeteria food was bland, calorie-laden gunk.

Not much time for partying but some looking for love in old places. The biggest crush of my young life—a friend's older brother. More than a crush, I felt high when with him. It must be love. We laughed, felt good around each other; had for years. A forbidden kiss snuck in times past, a phone call from him in California while I was just a high school senior. So what if he was older. Age doesn't stop feelings.

He was in law school in San Francisco. Came

unexpectedly one afternoon to my dorm for a visit. Another time took me out in the city dancing. Still felt high when around him, could not control my emotions. Met up one night for a few beers at a bar with his law school buddies, all older. How immature I must seem but I did paint my fingernails. And I did have a good sense of humor, was known to be smart. Did they think I would be a good match? Was I marriage material?

I was attractive, wasn't I? I could be the wife of an attorney. How much fun would that be? Where was my boyfriend? Why did nothing become anything of substance?

Then there was the slimy soccer coach (another European but nothing to write home about) who went big time for my pants but where was the conversation? We all need some physical affection but there was no connection. I wanted a relationship, to be close to someone. Wasn't drunken groping supposed to be just a preview, not the real thing?

High (though not on any drug) and erratic I got my roommate to go out partying. We went to a nice bar then back to a hotel with two men. They were older guys, maybe a bit too old but not too bad looking. Both doctors if not lying, in town for a conference they said. They were wearing suits.

Split into separate rooms with a daddy figure for each of us I couldn't go through with it. What was I doing? If I had been more experienced probably would have just given the blow job he was expecting and that would have been the end of that.

Instead, as he stood there with his pants belt unbuckled, I

laughed nervously; was feeling so uncomfortable. And I was worried about my friend. I was the one who got us into this fiasco I needed to be the one to get us out. Was she ok? I got me and my misled roomy out of there and back to our dorm room. Smarter than me in general, she'd declined the sex also. Think they just talked a bit.

Ok, now year three, this will be it. Why I played co-ed soccer on the weekends with friends who were engineering students and a mix of new guys and gals to hang out with. There has to be someone here who I would be interested in, who would be interested in me. Made more friends, did a little more dating yet was a pretty dry year all around. No wonder I was dispirited and feeling a little down.

To top it all off, a date for my 21st birthday to go see the band Heart in concert. I was asked out by the guy who lived in the apartment across the hall. He was a bit older, a blue collar type like the motorcycle guy who started off my college dating scene. Maybe I'd come full circle and this would be the one. He stood me up. And I also figured out was the one who was stealing my Sunday paper left out on the front door stoop weekly.

End of recap. This is where you think 'thank goodness this book is not about her sex life' or lack thereof and I get back to my writing about bipolar.

Where were we? Ah yes, clinical with The Drone...

And I was bipolar and taking medication via Dr. S and having to pay for those visits which was not easy at $100 a pop and having to take lithium which was causing excess

41

thirst and we thought possibly making the fatigue stuff worse so Dr. S took me off. And I was in clinical with The Drone who was making me, to say the least, feel uncomfortable. What had changed from the previous year?

The Drone had it out for me a bit, one morning having me go into a separate meeting room to talk. Weird? Yes, it was not normal, not a part of any of the required clinical work. And it wasn't friendly, The Drone was never cordial. It was like she started off the semester ready to target me. I never should have talked about my experience that occurred that summer, I was starting to realize.

The chat that I was required to have was about how women physicians have a high rate of suicide. Seriously. At the time I was whining about wanting to be a doctor rather than a nurse off and on; in private to any sympathetic slob who would listen, just working out my issues. I wasn't happy with school, none of my good friends were other nursing students and therefore is this really what I should be doing? I never went to the Pre-Med department and asked to enroll, I knew what my grades were.

I was also taking drawing classes at an Art Institute downtown during my free time and thinking of writing children's books.

That is what college years are supposed to be for. Before it became a way for the government and private investors to extort money out of individuals and public institutions and create a class of indentured servants; highly educated ones. A time for exploration, a chasing of one's dreams if you were lucky enough to know what those were. A time to try and

42

figure out career paths that would be a good fit for your talent and skills, no?

Guess not, at least for someone they knew was dealing with a mental illness. But again, what right did she have to pull me aside and talk to me about something she had no business talking to me about, much less the demoralizing, macabre way it was done? None.

In a way I was refusing to look at myself as anything less than what I was before the illness, or what I could have been even if I had no illness. Why shouldn't I? I was still a bright, caring human being who was allowed to have goals, aspirations and dreams. I really hadn't changed I was reinforcing to myself (though in an annoying way to others). Even though I was dealing with an illness it didn't mean I had no value or human worth.

The Drone kept on pulling whatever manipulative bullshit she could. When I had to miss a day of class for a university soccer game that was out of the city she arranged for it to be cause to visit the Dean of Nursing's office, I mean Queen C. Why? No reason, all athletes were allowed to play and not be penalized, make up coursework as needed. The Dean knew that very well, yet still had a little talk with me for much ado about nothing.

I didn't realize it at the time but they were beginning a pattern of harassment that would continue through the next semester until they finally figured out a way they could force me out of the program.

The 'Trio Three PhD's' did the harassment. All other

experiences I had with profs, graduate students teaching science labs, etc. were pretty run of the mill normal. I was an underperforming student (very unpredictable and inconsistent) but clearly bright and most seemed to like me. Or at least not show dislike. First I'd had of that was from The Drone.

I chose to go back to the university after Freshman Year and my grand debut into bipolar madness due to the kindness of the Physiology Professor, the graduate student guy who ran the lab and others. I could have gone running home in shame to never return but I felt that was a major cop out and what did I have to be ashamed of anyway?

Embarrassed? Of course. Even humiliated a little... and confused. Still wasn't quite sure what the heck had happened and what this new 'me' was all about.

But have I mentioned I also learned after coming out of that manic episode and going to the dorms with my mom to gather my things how friends had called looney bins for miles around to get to come and visit? I am sure they would have been drinking and considered it an adventure to escape the college doldrums like no other (grin)... but that isn't the point.

I had friends who were good people. I'd also spent a bunch of money and time already; it would have been a financial and personal loss to leave.

Finally time with The Drone ended, the semester was over. I had completed all the work, was given not great grades (could not possibly be that I was intentionally being graded down regardless of my performance) but passed. I thought I was done with The Drone but I was mistaken.

The harassment would not only continue, but get worse. After the holidays and start of the next semester I had to go and see The Drone for a talk. I had no idea why but was getting used to this crazy stuff pretty quickly.

It seems that a research paper I had completed and been given a passing grade for the previous semester (it was a bear of an assignment with time consuming research, I had to go to a medical library in the city to get reference material) was now considered an issue. Issue for what? I'd been given a grade, and a final grade in the class and a new semester was in progress. WTF?

I had to go to The Drone's office in the evening during a new semester full of more mindless but very time consuming coursework and days spent working at a hospital for these talks with The Drone on three or so occasions. The main inference was that somehow I had cheated the previous semester but I was never accused of cheating. Nothing was brought to my attention I could refute.

I hadn't, the paper was actually very well done. I was good at writing and had worked hard on the assignment.

The clinical rotation I was now in was General Medicine and the last one. The instructor was Nurse HeMan. Nurse HeMan, The Dean and The Drone were all friends and all had a doctorate degree in psychology from the UCSF graduate school.

After about three evening visits I arrived once again around 7 p.m., as directed to The Drone's office for what reason still was not clear. The Drone then told me I had to go and talk with Nurse HeMan whose office was just down the hall. Two minutes after I sat down wondering why I was there Nurse HeMan asked what medications I was taking. Just like that. Out of the blue, no reason for me to even be in her office.

The Drone's attempt to call me a plagiarizer was a bust, so this was their next little trick to pull.

Sadly, as I really wasn't processing how malicious in intent the actions of these women really were, I thought the question was being asked out of concern or curiosity. I had no shame in taking a prescribed medication for a diagnosed, treatable illness—concern about the illness but shame, no. I thought that since my reply was "lithium" and not "Thorazine", things would be ok. It wouldn't be long before I realized how wrong that assumption would prove to be.

It was inappropriate, violating and overtly manipulative but what was I to do? These women controlled my future at that point and I only wanted to be cooperative. I wasn't a combative, hostile person by nature. They had no business asking me about my medical history or any personal information for that matter, but especially not about medical information that is protected by law.

I was dismissed after they got the information they were after and—magically—the required visits that were never made clear why they were being required in the first place stopped.

From that point on I was a on a fast track to being forced out of the program. The harassment I was put through by these supposed 'health professionals' was calculated and relentless. And why? Simply because they knew I had received treatment for a mental illness. And now what medication I was taking, most likely asked as they wanted to know what diagnosis I had been given.

An experience with a patient flexing his muscle while I was giving a shot that subsequently caused a little blood to spurt out (I apologized profusely, he was undisturbed) became cause for a visit to The Dean's office. Nurse HeMan got the word 'gay' into a lecture and gave me a nice, long extended stare. Staring meant to make me feel uncomfortable and it did. So that is what this is all about, I would think afterwards. They are doing this as they think I am a lesbian?

Nurse HeMan was tall, unfeminine and brusque in manner. The irony is if there was any member of the nursing faculty batting for the team that would meet with disapproval by the high priests of the Catholic Church it was HeMan. Who these women were or were not spreading their legs for I could have cared less about; they seemed to be obsessed with me and my personal life.

Summer break was the light at the end of the tunnel. When this rotation was completed, I would have been eligible to take the state boards in the State of California and become a registered nurse. The last year in the four year baccalaureate nursing program I was in was a piece of cake compared to the grueling first three years, I was told by previous grads. Hang in there and get your degree.

They weren't breaking me, forcing me to possibly commit suicide from the harassment and added stress (or make an attempt that they knew would have caused me to leave the school) or drop out on my own. So they figured out a way to up the ante.

All of a sudden I was told that they did not have a current vaccination record on file for me. What? I was at the end of two years of work in hospitals yet two weeks before completing my final rotation they don't have my vaccination record that I had submitted Freshman Year? Why not?

Their efforts were now having results. I was getting near the breaking point. Again, I did what was required. I called my parents to have a new copy sent to the school, with my mom (now concerned as well) offering to fax one immediately. When I got upset at the records clerk asking why I was responsible for their negligence yet another meeting with The Dean was required where I was told I was being 'belligerent'.

I had never been called belligerent in my life. They refused to accept a fax and I just kept on doing what I had to do knowing I was almost done with having to deal with them for good.

"Not so fast, little one."

I got a phone call from Nurse HeMan the night before one of my last required days at the hospital. A few days more I was home free and would have survived what had turned into a hellish year. "You cannot attend clinical tomorrow," I was told, because they had no vaccination record on file for me.

The bomb had successfully and calculatedly been dropped. I had missed two days of clinical already because of my sports schedule and a week with the flu. You were only allowed three. Or maybe it was four, either way this forced absence put me over the allotted number. Their efforts concluded in the intended result. Another trip to The Dean's office and I was told "I had to withdraw". Finally I understood what was happening.

I was beyond myself with anger. I had spent an approximate $15,000 in loans for the semester and had no intention of repeating a semester—and paying another $15,000—that I had already completed assigned work for, including many hours caring for patients in hospital wards and outpatient settings.

What about having to pay for and attend childbirth classes before the OB/GYN semester? All those ugly white shoes and uniforms I had to buy and wear?

I would have had to have been psychotic to think of returning to the program the following year and have these same women be my university instructors. Masochism wasn't my thing. And if this was even an inkling of the type of community that makes up the nursing profession, I decided I would never have any part of it.

Nurse HeMan, The Drone and The Dean had all received doctorates in psychology from the University of California at San Francisco. UCSF clearly trained its graduates well in the art of malicious harassment of those given a psychiatric diagnosis. I had met my responsibilities under very difficult circumstances, they had repeatedly violated theirs. If anyone deserved sanctions it was them.

Maybe their doctorate indoctrination during their studies in regards to the segment of the population they were supposedly being trained in how to help was more of this nature: What should we do with these people? We can't kill them as then we will get into trouble, but we don't want to pay for them and they are not fit for work.

Not fit for work? We can move them into focused 'intentional communities' of sorts and then they will die off sooner naturally. Or will they? What if they don't, what then?

The hallowed halls of the University of San Francisco became known to me as POS.U—Piece of Shit University. I would have little other recourse as I was told by a 'friend of the family' lawyer when I wanted to sue for the calculated harassment I was subjected to and being forced to withdraw from the program, "No one is going to sue USF."

I didn't have the energy or willpower to contact anyone else. As someone young, not rich and dealing with a mental illness I was an easy victim.

Uncoded, the attorney's quick reply in support of the established institution without even hearing of what had transpired meant this: 'You have a mental illness, anyone can do what they want to you as far as society is concerned and experience no repercussions, because you are considered less than human. You do not have the same rights and protections granted other members of society.'

After I was forced out and moved back to Seattle I got a letter in the mail from POS.U asking for the reason why I had withdrawn. I clearly stated in my reply that I had not withdrawn at all, that I was forced to withdraw, told I had to. Shockingly, POS.U never replied back.

POS.U not only got away with it they reveled in their victory. The day I was told I 'had to withdraw' by The Dean I was not even invited into the office to sit down. I was met at the door and she was giddy with glee, happy to get to break the news. No, I am not being sarcastic.

I had been put into a category of having no dignity and worth, not worthy of any consideration. Of no value, someone it was 'ok' to harass and discriminate against. Someone it was ok to target.

CHAPTER 5

Mania & Hypomania

That fateful spring day of my Freshman Year I was transported from the crisis center (my first stop after the counselor's office at POS.U) to what seemed more like a drug rehabilitation facility for teenagers than psych ward. I was driven while strapped into the back of the fully enclosed and metal mesh reinforced van across the Bay Bridge and given a bed.

Only two things I really remember; being asked to call my parents and having a hysterical phone conversation and of having a reaction to one of the drugs. My parents were a bit freaked out as well. It seems they were never contacted when I first was deemed unable to care for myself and POS.U wasn't able to verify the insurance I had submitted upon enrolling.

Insurance meant for this exact type of thing; partly why I was being moved all over the place.

I was feeling very strange. I do not remember much except that I walked through the lounge area and then was led to my room by a staff member. It was late evening at this point and time for bed. The drug reaction was a new—it was all new that day and for many years after—feeling like an out-of-bounds anxiety that was taking myself hostage and that I had no control over.

The feeling of entering a mental nowhere land inside my brain that I would never return from.

It was beyond terrifying yet you have to lie there and let your cortical synapses do whatever the hell they feel like. You have no control over anything. Not the state you are in, not the drugs you will be instructed to take, not your system's response or lack of response to the medications. Everything is completely out of your control.

My mom had flown in from out of town and used to say that night was the scariest for her as well; she sensed the same thing. I do remember her coming in the room, and I do remember lying there completely helpless. I do remember knowing how she felt, that she knew something was seriously wrong with her daughter yet she was an experienced nurse (a very good one) and played that role along with mother; calm touch, calm voice, telling me to rest.

Luckily I was able to sleep. They stopped drugging me and by the next morning the extreme emotional states and feelings for the most part went away. I wasn't in terror land anymore and hoped to never return. The attending psychiatrist—a distinguished looking, friendly, older guy—came into the breakfast room to say hello. After seeing my progress, and that I could actually communicate like a normal person again, he pronounced me sane enough to head home.

That's Dr. S whom I've mentioned already. The S as in

'savior' as that is what it felt like he was at that moment in time. He wasn't forcing me to take any additional medications or having me carted off somewhere else. I was being allowed to leave. I liked Dr. S.

If you have never been drugged—voluntarily or involuntarily—it is an experience that is hard to explain. During 30 years of living with this illness I have only experienced this state four or five times, all during an episode of mania that had progressed into psychosis.

If you have willingly been psychotic i.e. taken recreational hallucinogenic drugs for the fun of it, you may have an idea of what it is like. When it occurs outside of your control and without choice, it is a terrifying experience.

I usually do not hear voices or see things that are not there. One time I did go into 'another world' of sorts and was completely psychotic. Much more to it than this little fragment but for a part of it I entered into a jungle environment with real live beasts communicating with me. There were lions roaring, tigers snarling, other larger than life unworldly creatures invading my consciousness.

I know that sounds strange (whatever form psychosis takes it is usually strange) and yes it was but these things were not just being 'imagined'. I was mentally there with them knowing it wasn't real yet was being experienced in my mind as completely real. And it was terrifying. I ended up leaving jungle land to walk somewhere though had no idea where I was going. I had no shoes on and did not know why or where they were.

The police picked me up as I was trying to make a phone call from a payphone. I knew on some level it was a good thing they put me in the back of the squad car but when they drove into the enclosed garage space with adjoining door to their holding cell area the internal fear I was experiencing amplified through the roof. What are they going to do to me?

At this stage of the game you are not aware that you are having an episode. You are just mentally out of it and scared out of your skull.

I had just moved in with a guy I didn't know well (platonic roommate kind-of thing) and a little before I went into this manic psychosis I'd eaten and drunk something out of the fridge. It is possible I was drugged. LSD? The whole thing happened so quickly and was unlike any other high state of my illness. When he came into the house and saw me lying on broken glass on the couch (from a painting hanging on the wall I had felt compelled to break) he just looked at me unsurprisingly. I was obviously confused and out of it yet he said nothing. He did not ask if I was ok or what had happened.

If I had been drugged unknowingly—for whatever reason or purpose—he was the one the police should have taken to their holding cell scared out of their wits. And then booked, charged with criminal assault and hopefully successfully prosecuted. The little piss ant.

Most persons understanding of psychosis is from Hollywood movie portrayals or literary stereotypes and usually is of someone with the mental illness schizophrenia. The psychosis of mania is more akin to having your normal self—that person you wake up and live with 24/7 for most days of your life—be overtaken by emotions that have spun out of control. Your body (and mind) has gone into hyperdrive without you pushing any button or pulling any lever. Hang on tight as things could get rough.

You are out of control yet there is no reason why it should be happening. You did nothing to cause it yet chemical processes in your brain have switched operating systems without your consent. The wallpaper they are slapping up on your neurons for you to view and experience in your mental browser is the Crazyland theme.

And I was very content with the rolling brook scene, soft Jazz music playing in the background, thank you very much. Last week's view of the Eiffel Tower and rowdy tourists drinking, partying it up in the grass late at night, a couple off to the side having a little tryst wasn't so bad either. But this Crazyland theme? I never chose this.

Here is a physical analogy to the mental state of mania. You eat a lot of fattening foods, don't exercise and put on weight. Say maybe a pound or two. That is normal and expected. But going manic is like you woke up one morning and your body was not your body... it's HUGE, unrecognizable in the mirror to you or anyone who knows you in your normal physical state. And how the heck did that happen?

You did nothing to cause it... ok, maybe an extra bag of Lays and a few too many cupcakes, skipped the gym on Tuesday.

You cannot fit into your pants, you can hardly walk.

Can't go to work as how would you fit in that office chair? Why worry about going to work, you have to find a tailor stat. No store in the universe sells pants to cover that humongous backend, they may even have to invent a new form of zipper.

Meanwhile your internal self is trying to talk, still trying to relate if it can. What happened? What did I do to cause this? Then reality sets in. It does not matter that you did nothing to cause this massive body change which is beyond any norm most other persons would experience, there it is and you have to deal with it.

I have only experienced psychosis on a few occasions, none of which were due to my ingesting psychoactive substances but from my body going into a manic state during a period of rapid cycling. And thankfully my particular version of this genetically-based disease responds to medications available for treatment.

To put it another way… the few times I have had to be hospitalized, I have been released within two weeks or less as was able to stabilize quickly.

The episode goes something like this. I flip, start to escalate, stand out from the crowd a bit, just a tad, especially when causing a major disturbance and then spiral out of control. Like the time I ranted in the streets of downtown Seattle about PhDs (I really did and yes, it was connected to POS.U) or when an uncle happened to call my parents and I answered giving out a nasty rant about 'T-Shirt' businesses.

Yes, T-Shirts. And this person was the nicest you'd want to meet, a father to a large crew of my cousins with constant

Irish twinkle in his eye and rosy-red nose to go with it. He was always kind and caring to me whenever we exchanged the customary hellos at a family gathering (holidays, wedding). Crazy? Yes. In a 'hypomanic on the verge of mania' state? Check.

And btw, in case you are new to this, if there is anything we need to all be in uproar about on this planet (this was in 1993 or 1994 maybe they've made changes in the industry) it is those darn T-Shirt vendors!

I was a bit mortified as I had no idea where the rant came from and apologized soon after, kind of like an alcoholic who has to make amends to those they hurt while under the influence. Just because I was hypomanic does not mean I didn't have responsibility for my actions.

Lucky for me it is rare that my high states involve lashing out at others. I am usually laughing, laughing, laughing and it is all very funny until it isn't. Or getting busy, busy, busy until whatever it is I am so busy with (but rarely getting much done) turns into me being one of the busiest people within miles and a switch to craziness ensues.

Like the time I got on a plane to San Francisco while finishing a degree years later at the University of Washington (1997) and needed an escape. I had to do something. My brain and body wanted to move, to go, to be somewhere, do something. Off the plane (don't recall a lot of it now) somehow wandering around I ended up in a little deli and hung out, then made a new friend: the owner.

He was extra-social—matched my state of mind very

well—attractive (dark and a bit mysterious) and attracted to me. He invited me to go to a pub for a bite to eat and what else did I have to do but nothing. Of course I had not planned this grand adventure much in advance. I did not even know where I would sleep that night.

Laughing, laughing, laughing, could not stop laughing. He was cute and trying hard to be charming, getting a huge kick out of this wayward gal he picked up that thought just about anything he said was worthy of a new round of giggles. Energy all around, we drove around the city, did some touristy things then—surprise—went back to his apartment.

A couple massage exchanges, nice night of mutually gratifying erotic tussle between the sheets and then the hangover starts to lift in the morning. Shit. What have I done and why am I here? Weekend not over, another night stay and I almost got to play pool with Don Johnson—yes, THE Don Johnson… how cool would that have been?

The guy was a bit of a mover and shaker, took me to a movie set thing going on (all I remember is food, think he may have been part of the catering team) and then later was invited to go hang out and play pool somewhere. Whether Don J. would have been there or not, have no idea. Around 4 p.m. that afternoon I started to crash back down a bit and realized how strange it was what I was doing, where I was.

And I hadn't packed to hang with a movie star. Wear these jeans and this shirt, again? If I drink a couple of beers will I feel good, like I can take on the universe and go anyways? No, just got tired and to bed early I went, with cute pick up guy getting me to the airport the next morning. Back at the ranch (this time in Seattle) never spoke of the episode to anyone.

Back on my bike the next morning and off to class, back to the college stress that I was handling well by taking only two classes instead of the usual three and enjoying much. Stimulating coursework in New Media, Communications and Journalism that I took to easily, sharp professors whom I respected and decent grades finally.

The memory of the whole escapade faded fast but it is probably the most successful (and was fun) hypomanic state I have ever been in; clearly on the verge of mania but didn't flip. That kind of thing usually isn't very successful for BP-1 folks like me.

I usually cannot stop the derailed train of a brain (mine) going at that speed.

CHAPTER 6

Hospitalizations & Getting Better

If I start to cycle into the high end of the bipolar mood spectrum it rarely is fun for very long, though hypomanic states can be very fun. My version of this mood disorder plays out on high volume, with the brain veering off the tracks and the 'choo choo' fading into the distance quickly. I fly off those tracks!

Rather than a crazy, fun time I end up hospitalized where I am drugged and crash back down to normal—usually within a day or so. Normal in the sense of no more psychosis.

My normal self returns albeit a bit ragged from the experience and there I sit. Hanging out on the ward, taking meds, eating nasty, processed food meals (you do not know what the term glutinous means until you have been served a plate of this chow) and doing a few casual things like naps and attempts at reading.

Staying put until I am legally able to be released back into the realm of human living.

Socializing isn't big on the wards but there are some very social co-inmates at times, just those are usually the ones you need to steer clear of. Jibber jabber, jibber jabber and maybe a look in your direction… eeks, look away, look away. Or that jibber jabber may get directed at you and sometimes what they say is not very nice.

One time it was a roommate, who then threatened to stab me with a knife. Thankfully my request to be relocated to a room down the hall was granted. The new roomy was experiencing major depression and reading her bible quietly non-stop; a nice person to share with and exchange hellos, 'how are you doing'.

Another time my roommate thought I was a doctor. Really. There I was, sitting on the bed across the room from her as I had been for the previous day and a half and she asked me if I was one of the physicians. Sure, I am Dr. Molly and thought I would don a gown and hang with my homies, the patients.

Er, no. I am in here for the same reasons you are I assured her, then helped her make her bed. I felt a little bad for her if she was that out of it. I had already cleared out of my craziness.

This gal, unlike me, had wanted to be admitted but another facility she went to refused. What did she do? She got in a car and tried to storm the place by attempting to drive through the front door. No one was hurt, the staff member who had to jump out of the way did not press charges and she got her way (though car keys taken away). She was admitted to the same ward I was in; my new temporary friend and roommate.

Only once did one incarceration lead to a second one not

long after as the medication I was prescribed to take and did as directed ended up creating more chemical imbalance. The sad reality is as much as psychotropic drugs can be useful in managing mental illness, or like in my case at least alleviate its severe states, they are toxic substances.

Toxic chemical compounds that can trigger rapid cycling, worsening of whatever state you are in or a flip to the other side of the mood coin.

I can remember clearly the afternoon it started. I was still sane but starting to have some psychotic symptoms. I smelled smoke and could not figure out where it was coming from. I checked all through my parents' condo and no smoke to be seen, no fire.

Out on the balcony I went... is there something going on outside that I am smelling? No. Back in the house I go and I still smell the smoke, sitting at the kitchen table near the phone; I smell smoke! Where is it coming from and I need to figure this out now so that I can call the fire department.

Still smell smoke. I feel the wall and lean in close, touching the wall to see if I could feel any heat coming from the other side... maybe that apartment is on fire! I either went next door and knocked or banged on the wall, but low and behold all was well.

One of the nice, young, good-looking (of course) firefighters out of about five who happened to live there (yes, true story) checked things out and assured me all was well. If there was a problem, those guys would have had it covered.

Now as opposed to saving the day I was very

embarrassed. I started to process what was going on from an internal angle. No smoke but a strong smell of it triggering my brain to think there is a fire. What is actually going on is an olfactory hallucination. Simply put, I was smelling something that wasn't there.

The one and only time in my life I've experienced such a thing, an experience caused by a psychotropic medication.

Great. Just what I needed to make my day and yes, did I not just take a little pill a little bit before all this occurred, out of that saffron-brown shaded plastic bottle that is right in front of me on the kitchen table? Has my name on the white label. Yep, that's it.

Yet another medication in the good doc's arsenal who was trying to help me stabilize that was found to be not only useless, but creating dangerous side effects. Then comes all the stress of what to do next.

Just as the legal system is in large part about protecting the property—in all its guises—of the wealthy, psychiatry functions as a safeguard for society against persons who are mentally ill. And in many cases the two work in conjunction with each other.

The four times I was involuntarily hospitalized two things occurred. First I was deemed a threat to either myself or others (in my case always myself due to severe depression or mania that had spiraled out of control) and the second is I stay an approximate two weeks, sleep lots, ingest chemical substances (pink or white pills, sometimes blue), eat shitty food and then it is adios time.

"Have fun, be good out there little one."

To be admitted for an involuntary stay you attend a hearing, have an attorney present and receive a commitment order from a judge. As I am not a big fan of psych wards it was always involuntary in my case. And just because I am a non-violent person who does as she is asked in that type of situation doesn't mean I didn't cause a bit of a ruckus at times; I did.

The time I thought I was going to be zapped with ECT while waiting strapped onto a gurney to be taken to where they had a bed available was one time I took a while to stabilize. When I was finally transported and admitted to the ward at the assigned location I was still pretty high. And my self was very unhappy to have been put in that situation. "It's not fair," she ranted.

And she—I mean I—ranted for hours at the window. Moaned more than ranted really, saying over and over again in a low, monotonous tone, "No trial." "No trial, no trial," I said to anyone who may have been walking outside on the sidewalk below and heard me. Like they would have filed a petition with the court or staged a public protest on my behalf.

'It's just a looney bin patient,' any in-the-know neighbors would have registered.

My inner self at the time was pissed. "What the heck have I done to deserve this," she questioned. Then went on, "No trial…" An hour or so later whatever med I had been given kicked in and I fell fast asleep. Knocked out cold sleep, exactly what I needed.

I remember waking up once during the night as my sleeping subconscious sensed something in the room. Eyes opened with fear, then relaxed. A hospital staff member was sitting quietly in a chair near the end of the bed. Felt peaceful and calming, most likely she was in silent prayer. Or at least sneaking a break by putting her feet up for a bit after having to come and check on me.

When five years or more pass after an episode I always fall into the trap of thinking I've been cured. The illness has somehow permanently gone away and I will not have to deal with it anymore.

What bipolar illness? What psychiatric hospitalizations?

The previous experiences fade into the distant background of my psyche and are rarely recalled. Other issues come to the forefront, normal ones like work, staying fit, trying to have a bit of fun. Just not too much fun and be careful if you start laughing too hard or too loudly...

When the illness returns in one form or another I am forced to acknowledge its existence. Everything else—those regular things—gets put aside. Once again I become a person with a mental illness who needs treatment, not the normal functioning being of the months and years prior.

It's back to non-human, subhuman status.

CHAPTER 7

Playing Doctor Roulette

The summer after being kicked out of college was uneventful yet not without a few highlights. It was nice to connect with a few old high school friends, be in a familiar place and do a little healthy partying and fraternizing; the usual stuff. I rented a room in a shared house with a few others also back in the area after attending out-of-state schools and found a job.

I landed one of the wondrous low-paying jobs so abundantly available to a 21 year old with a lot of work experience but no college degree. Getting paid a little over minimum wage while my student loan debt bills started to arrive in the mail.

On the other front was incorporation into the medical model of mental illness yet even the first psychiatrist who treated me—Dr. S—recommended other illnesses be ruled out such as mononucleosis or a sleep disorder. Did I have a brain tumor?

After a foot operation in high school (gifted surgeon, four hours, 19 pieces of glass removed, a few different colors of glass they told me) I had a slightly turned in right foot and strange new propensity to use my left hand though am right-handed. I had difficulty completing schoolwork and had to retrain myself how to run i.e. my turned-in foot kept throwing me off balance, making me almost trip.

I also started to take naps before sports games as would become so sleepy in the afternoon—strange for any healthy, active 16 year old. Had I suffered a minor stroke? Did a nurse miss an air bubble in an IV?

To lessen the blow of my newly diagnosed condition I was told how "lucky" I was to be one of the few diagnosed with Manic Depression that has been suffered by some of society's greatest; many hardworking, successful business persons, engineers, artists, politicians, musicians etc. At one point even that it was a status symbol (that was Dr. H whom you will meet below).

Unfortunately, it is not the type of status most young adults are searching for or are comfortable with.

Our family physician suggested I see the psychiatrist my mom had seen weekly for around 15 years. The one my mom saw on the side. It was a secret of sorts. When in high school I was asked to not talk to my father about it and I never did. My mother was never seriously ill—physically or mentally—just a person in life needing some outside care to deal with the stresses of her life.

She did not take psychotropic medications yet humorously told the tale of how she was put on Ritalin once as an adult (as a nurse, she knew that was a bit odd). In her mid-twenties she was given thyroid hormone to help conceive after a few years of marriage and no bundles of joy to fuss over. It worked; five of them materialized in the years that followed.

She did take the commonly prescribed at the time 'stressed-out housewife and mother' pill: valium. She took it on occasion to help get a good night's rest. She never smoked. Drank a drink or two on a holiday or at a special event but for all practical purposes was a teetotaller.

My dad was a regular drinker and the 'fun Dad' type of drinker. He owned his own insurance business and we lived comfortably middle class. As he aged he drank more and was an alcoholic. And not so much fun. My mom could never understand it. One alcoholic beverage gave her a mild hangover the next day. She didn't enjoy alcohol. My dad self-medicated with it.

He also smoked when I was a young child. Then his precious offspring revolted over the revolting smell and made him quit. Cigars were his thing. Family birthday photos of that time usually involved a photograph of him, a cigar case and a smile.

The doctor it was recommended I have an evaluation with was one of the cutest psychiatrists you'd ever want to meet. I'll nickname him Dr. H with the 'H' standing for Hobbit even though the movie hadn't been out yet. Very short and small in stature, pretty old and odd-looking but you knew in a heartbeat a top notch, caring person. We chatted, he shared the story of his breakdown of sorts during his first year of medical school where his friends locked him in a closet until he calmed down; not nice.

A devout Catholic he went on to finish his schooling, have a family and be one of the brave souls to care for other souls who may not be so brave or who have been dealt a difficult set of genetic cards. I told my 'story' again to Dr. H (got sick of that really quickly as the months and years went on) of what I had experienced.

He listened, asked a few questions and performed a brief exam of my neck, checking for enlarged lymph nodes. Chronic Fatigue Syndrome (now also called Myalgic Encephalomyelitis or ME) was coming onto the scene and I had complained of fatigue and daytime drowsiness for years.

He told me about a sharp, young doctor he knew whom he thought would be able to help. At the end of the short chat session I impulsively gave him a hug. I was happy to get to walk out of there but also as Dr. H was such a sweetheart and had been so kind, went out of his way to ease my anxieties.

On to the next doc. Let's call him 'Sexy 2' with tall, dark and handsome sleep specialist doc that he would work with closely during my care fitting the 'Sexy 1' profile. Both physicians were good looking, smart, young, ambitious, accomplished doctors in their fields and I knew I was lucky to be their patient.

I was a psychiatric patient and for that reason alone who knew what would happen to me or what I would be subjected to. My experience at POS.U had taught me that; to fear, be afraid of what others in positions of power may do since I had been labeled mentally ill.

Sexy 2 was a nice guy and we had a good rapport.

Unfortunately for me and my care Sexy 2 had a theory and I was manipulated a bit into being one of his guinea pigs. It was a pretty easy sell. I had an illness, was young, naive, needed treatment and was clueless as to what that treatment was or should be other than needing to take medications.

CHAPTER 8

The Lithium Cure That Didn't Work

Sexy 2 wanted me to take high doses of lithium for a year. I had taken lithium in college for a few months but the side effects made me go off. Now with Sexy 2 at the helm lithium treatment was not only back on the table it was seen as the primary form of treatment my form of bipolar illness needed; the granddaddy of them all, Bipolar I Disorder.

He let me know the lithium he was prescribing would require monthly blood monitoring. And that we would meet once a week. I was fine with all of it. I simply wanted to be a good patient, chat with Sexy 2 as was required and take whatever drug I was told to. I wanted to be well, to not cause my family, self or anyone else distress and get on with my life.

He was a good guy Sexy 2. He had an attractive wife who was a RN (crossed paths in the office waiting room), two young children at the time and used to play soccer in college. I was a bit enamored even though the visits and chats were mandatory and knew it was his professional role to be a bit charming. Did I mention the sexy voice? Calm, soothing, sort-of rough around the edges…

Sexy 1's role was to make sure I did not have an actual sleep disorder or other related medical condition. That I really was 'just' bipolar and needed to be treated that way. Or possibly be given a dual diagnosis of bipolar and a sleep disorder.

They were simply being very thorough and trying to identify causes of the fatigue and daytime drowsiness (almost to the point of nodding off) I suffered from. Making sure the symptoms were caused by a clinical depression and bipolar related.

Many physical illnesses can mimic symptoms of depression and even cause psychosis. Sexy 1 took a very detailed history, worked with Sexy 2 in prescribing any medications (so as not to push me over a manic ledge) and did testing for narcolepsy. I spent an afternoon at his high tech sleep lab but all was found to be fine. Back to my primary care provider Sexy 2 I went.

The theory Sexy 2 had that I had become a test subject for unknowingly was to evaluate if giving Bipolar I patients (the most serious form of the illness) lithium in high doses over a year's time would 'cure' cyclic depression and mania. Meaning it would cycle a rapid cycling patient out of major depression and out of serious mania. Turn a BP-1 sufferer more into a Bipolar II Disorder (BP-2) state.

I am pretty sure that was the general idea.

He was just prescribing a form of chemical lobotomy i.e. saturating brain cells with high amounts of a toxic substance for a period of time hoping that it would change their chemical disposition or functioning. He was basically trying to affect mania, so that BP-1 sufferers like me would have less serious manic episodes. That would in turn affect the depressive swing of the cycle as it seemed to correlate to the severity of the manic period.

At that time in the mid 80s the awareness of mixed states and rapid cycling was just beginning to be identified. And keeping BP-1 patients out of mania and major depressive episodes would have been a heroic feat; as well I am sure in some circles of sufferers and their treatment providers even today.

Rapid-cycling Bipolar Disorder is described on the *National Institute of Mental Health (NIMH)* website as follows:

"A severe form of the disorder is called Rapid-cycling Bipolar Disorder. Rapid cycling occurs when a person has four or more episodes of major depression, mania, hypomania, or mixed states, all within a year."

"Rapid cycling seems to be more common in people who have their first bipolar episode at a younger age. One study found that people with rapid cycling had their first episode about four years earlier—during the mid to late teen years— than people without rapid cycling bipolar disorder. Rapid cycling affects more women than men. Rapid cycling can come and go."

Source: What is Bipolar Disorder?

http://www.nimh.nih.gov/health/publications/bipolar-disorder-in-adults/index.shtml?rf=

Bipolar II Disorder depressive and high states of the illness are a big step down from what Bipolar I persons and those who require frequent hospitalization experience. BP-2 patients have hypomanic episodes that us BP-1 folks think are a joy compared to manic episodes (or at least I do). I sure as heck have never complained about one.

Add rapid cycling to this mix and it is the proverbial hell on earth to live through, especially if a sufferer is unresponsive to treatment like I was at the time.

In explanation, think of running down a train track a bit haphazardly as it is summer and you feel free, the sunlight shining down, warm on your face making you feel happy and full of life. You may wave your arms a bit impulsively at any passersby but are being careful to some extent to watch for any impending locomotive.

You are acting a little erratic and lose track of time but are just having an exceptionally great day; a bit crazy but fun time.

Now visualize what a true manic episode might look like. No running, running is for imbeciles. You are flying, flying free, moving upwards towards the sun. You can feel the heat on your face, penetrating your skin, your body moving in sync with the rays of light that are reflecting off the shiny metal tracks; you are free, you will always be free. Nothing will stop you and nothing can stop you. Not even an advancing locomotive.

"Chugga chugga..." What's that? "Choo choo... ". I don't care, hit me, just try and hit me. I am invincible. Nothing can hurt me. I am free.

That was probably the realistic goal he was setting; to treat my illness to the extent it would be manageable and I would not require hospitalization. To eradicate mania in hopes it eradicated some of the mood cycling and I would suffer lesser (or at least fewer with more time lapse in between) high states.

He was trying to lessen the sensitivity of those overactive cell receptors some so my high states would reach heights more akin to the hypomania of Bipolar II as opposed to the manic psychosis of Bipolar I Disorder I knew all too well.

Unfortunately it was not a success. I was in treatment for major depression that did initially improve but then only got worse leading to a few visits with conversations about the inpatient facility at the hospital. Nope, that I was going to do all in my power—even if it meant suicide—to prevent.

I was becoming disillusioned as a patient, and frustrated that I seemed to not be improving much though was repeatedly told "things will get better". The promise all health care providers want to be able to offer their patients—follow the prescribed treatment and your symptoms or illness will improve or be cured. But that wasn't happening.

The main problem was that the lithium made me tired and fatigue was already a major symptom. The antidepressants I would try over the course of that year to combat this fatigue all had adverse effects and had to be stopped.

A tricyclic antidepressant helped for a bit. I had less fatigue and drowsiness, felt normal and started to get hopeful

I would have a future. The good docs who were trying hard to make my treatment a success had found something that was working. I had become cautious at this point to not get my hopes up for anything to be a permanent fix.

Bipolar I Disorder does not play out that way and I was learning the game quickly. Yet I was still young, naive and felt that way anyways. Maybe that's all I needed... a little dose of this antidepressant, stay on the lithium and life would be happy ever after after all.

Didn't happen. I started to have heart palpitations and had to go off of it. Heart palpitations can be an early physical sign of an impending manic episode—that full-on body speeding up where you don't have the options of pressing any brake pedal. And most likely require hospitalization, major doses of medication and more destruction to the little bit of self-esteem I was still hanging on to after POS.U.

Neither Sexy 1, Sexy 2 nor I wanted that to happen.

During my prescribed high-dosage/over-dosage of lithium spree my hair went curly. After a trip to a walk-in stylist for the usual trim my waves turned into thick, trundled masses of curls. No telling what havoc large amounts of psychotropic meds will play on your body.

When asked whether I had gotten a perm what was I supposed to say? That no, but I was on mega doses of lithium and maybe that was the cause even though up to that time it would have been a yet unheard of side effect?

At times I thought the Gods were having a good time messing with me. I, on the other hand, was spending very little time being amused.

Later after ending my time with Sexy 2 and slowly getting off the lithium and feeling a bit better, I was angry that I was used; or thought I had been used. I wanted to sue Sexy 2 for malpractice, yada yada... Bipolar I type of folks you really don't want to piss off.

I may look at it differently now, 27 years later, but know at the time the anger was not only legitimate, it was healthy. When the high doses of lithium were causing an increase in fatigue and a resultant increase in serious depression the dose should have been lowered to see if symptoms would lessen, not keep me on it to try and prove some theory.

I was a paying patient, not a clinical drug study subject.

CHAPTER 9

Bipolar Disorder vs Drug Addiction

A friend was worried about a friend. He went three days snorting coke with no sleep... again, and was out of control. Then he gets really depressed, she said. She told me he was bipolar. Not meaning to be unsympathetic yet most likely sounding exactly that I said bullshit. That the street drugs were just creating an illusion of it.

Or the 'bullshit' may have been my inner dialogue. I think I was a bit more polite in the actual conversation.

Why so unsympathetic? Was I being egotistical and self-centered in my thinking, a bipolar diagnosis snob of sorts? Yes. But the real underlying issue was that I was jealous. Twenty-four years old at the time and trapped in the eye of the bipolar hurricane (shit storm?) that had taken over my life, I was very jealous of others—all those normal folks who were not forced to live with a mental illness.

I wanted to be a hipster like the cool gals I was staying with at the time who could party hard, suffer a bit the day after but function in society and get to move forward in their lives, have control over their lives. The fun-loving, charismatic chicks who were talking about a friend of theirs as we chatted in the kitchen of the small apartment while preparing a meal and sharing a few beers.

I was not only jealous, but also completely oblivious to the extent that drug addiction can be connected to the illness of bipolar. I understood how street drugs (and certain prescription medications) could trigger an episode of mania leading to psychosis and that the person may then be diagnosed with underlying bipolar illness.

That I got clearly as it was similar to my personal experience.

What I had no clue about was the number of people who may suffer with a less severe form of bipolar (or other mental illness such as depression) and use drugs to self-medicate. I say 'less severe' as it would be unusual to not get identified as mentally ill if you have Bipolar I Disorder. Hard to not be hospitalized in a psychiatric facility at some point as well.

Self-medicating an undiagnosed mental disorder makes perfect sense. Their addiction is connected to the underlying biochemical imbalance that had not been identified or treated. A fancy term used by mental health professionals is 'comorbid substance abuse' and the patient is given a dual diagnosis of both drug addiction and bipolar illness.

The below information describing this connection is quoted from the website *Dual Diagnosis.org*:

"Like substance abuse, bipolar disorder poses a risk to the individual's physical and emotional well-being. Those afflicted with bipolar disorder have a higher rate of relationship problems, economic instability, accidental injuries and suicide than the general population. They are also significantly more likely to develop an addiction to drugs or alcohol."

Source: Bipolar Disorder and Addiction

http://www.dualdiagnosis.org/bipolar-disorder-and-addiction/

But it is also important to note and acknowledge not all bipolar sufferers are addicts. In fact, not being on drugs or a drug addict is one of the criteria used in the DSM-5 (Fifth Edition of the Diagnostic and Statistical Manual of Mental Disorders) to diagnose bipolar illness.

If you had a psychosis as a result of taking illegal drugs or experience depression or an irritable mood during a withdrawal phase you would most likely be given the diagnosis "Substance-Induced Mood Disorder", not bipolar. There are nine categories of Substance-Induced Disorders.

A brief explanation of illnesses in this category is quoted from the *Substance Abuse and Mental Health Services Administration (US)* below:

"Substance-induced disorders are distinct from independent co-occurring mental disorders in that all or most of the psychiatric symptoms are the direct result of substance use. This is not to state that substance-induced disorders preclude co-occurring mental disorders, only that the specific symptom cluster at a specific point in time is more likely the result of substance use, abuse, intoxication, or withdrawal than of underlying mental illness."

Source: National Center for Biotechnology Information,

I was so snippy about the issue in my younger years as I was not a drug abuser, active physically and always healthy yet I became ill. I had no control over the onset of illness that had developed within my brain. I drank alcohol off and on to have a good time, but never took street drugs except ecstasy once, at the beach, with a group of people I was living with at the time.

Yes, it was a cool experience. And on the rare occasion a little weed. And that was that. I knew I could not play around with any of that stuff or would flip out.

After being diagnosed I understood this about myself and about the illness. In not doing these things and accepting that I cannot do them I maintain a level of control and affect the incidences of crisis I experience. And some control over the inevitable suicidal depressions that would follow the high state.

To just view either illness—addiction or bipolar—in terms of an overabundance of this or an under-abundance of that is oversimplified and a bit of a cop-out. Any illness is partly an expression of self, whether physical or mental in origin. The person hosting the illness has some culpability, some personal connection to its causes and effects.

And if that is the case to some extent, then it can be empowering to believe you have some control over the experience. Not complete control but some ability to effect change i.e. to make things better or worse. To take some responsibility for your illness and not just rely on factors outside your control such as how medications may or may not work, what treatments are available during your lifetime, cravings for drugs or alcohol, etc.

Don't entrust your mental wellness or sobriety to others; learn to rely more on your inner resources, internal control.

If I was a drug user I would most likely be severely ill at this moment, unable to write a letter much less a book. If I had acted out the desire I had at times during my younger years (becoming a single Mom and working full-time ended that silliness) to have more fun, get crazy, party hard, stay up all night, live it up as you never know when you are going to die... most likely I would have been hospitalized many more than the four times I was.

And who knows what else may have happened. I could have possibly triggered a trip into the psych void to never return, never function in society again. That was the dark-grey, bleak, vaporless cloud hanging over my head for many years, following me wherever I went—that I would never improve only get worse.

In San Francisco cocaine was always available (and offered) and I wanted to try it but knew I couldn't. If a little speed had helped send me over the edge I could only imagine what snorting coke would do. Dr. S had actually made a point of warning me as well, to never touch the stuff and I knew he DID know what it would do.

That was probably half of his patient load; substance abusers with mental problems. The other half possibly consisting of mentally ill persons who abuse substances.

The below is from an article on *The Ranch – A Substance Abuse Treatment Facility* website:

"The frequency with which individuals who have bipolar disorder also suffer from substance abuse is very high. In fact, it leaves little doubt that there is a link between the two although it is not yet known which condition leads to the other. It is estimated that approximately 60% of all individuals with bipolar disorder also abuse substances."

Source: Bipolar Disorder and Substance Abuse

http://www.recoveryranch.com/articles/dual-diagnosis/bipolar-disorder-substance-abuse/

But not all bipolar sufferers abuse drugs and have the option of abstaining from an action or activity in order to get well. Like many others with Bipolar I Disorder my brain went awry in and of itself. Drug abusers have a choice to use or not use.

If you snort cocaine, pop acid or ecstasy, shove a needle in your arm, go on a binge, can't handle the drug load you have willingly inflicted upon your body and end up in a psych ward for a manic or other type of psychosis, you're an addict.

Get off the drugs and most likely you'll be fine. Bipolar illness sufferers do not have that choice. Behavior modification or will power worthy of an Olympic athlete is not going to cure the disease. You may remain symptom free for long periods of time depending on the type and severity of the illness but can never claim victory over its presence.

That is what made me so stuck-up in my thinking at the

time: anger over having my choices limited, my freedom living in the world curtailed. Some bastard process in my brain had changed my state of existence and there was nothing I could do about it, no way to revert the process. I simply had to learn to live with it.

Unlike a drug addict abstaining from their substance of choice the normal, functioning self of the bipolar could, can and most likely will be hijacked at any time, many times during the person's life, with or without outside contributing factors.

The insensitive 'who's better or worse', 'us vs them' attitude can go both ways; or at least the need to separate one from the other depending on which side you are on. Those who are bipolar and do suffer from addiction—dual diagnosis folks—are of course different and have a heavier load to carry. I emphasize with that situation greatly.

Alcohol is my drug of choice, and I've had to assess my use a few times during the past years, both on a personal level and with care providers.

I'm not an addict, but I do at this time in my life drink red wine almost daily and do find it helps much with many health issues, including my bipolar illness. I also have fibromyalgia from a mugging years back and it helps keep pain down, stress manageable and my muscles relaxed for deep sleep at night. Not to mention I deserve a little pleasure in my life.

During a period of successful remission when I've been free of the extreme states of being associated with this illness i.e. major, debilitating depression and mania of a BP-1 diagnosis as well as the life interrupting lite versions (hypomania and moderate depression) I visited my brother in a drug rehab facility.

I'd completed a college degree (albeit years late and just shy of 30 years old), was Mom to a healthy, very bright child who was well cared for and loved and had a good-paying job in the high tech field. Without the disease interfering for an extended time my life was able to move forward and progress in a way many others take for granted.

Walking through the facility with my parents and young son we were led to a back area where the patients were hanging-out taking a break. My brother was among them, along with a visiting friend of his who began entertaining my son with a football. We were just being there, present, showing support and care.

Someone was missing from the group and the jokes started that maybe he'd defected to the looney bin up the street. Those people were really sad cases, obviously... ones to one-up, help yourself feel better by berating.

I highly doubt the 'loonies' up the street were sitting around cracking jokes about the druggies down the road, but no matter. I couldn't believe I was there to offer support, and ended up getting inadvertently slammed. It seems you can never get away from it, no matter how well you do, what your good intentions are.

CHAPTER 10

Relapse, Suicide Risk & Times Past

You think you're well and you are. Moving along, living life, working, relating to others... then the change happens. One way or the other, highs or lows or a combination of the two the illness returns. Out of the blue or with weeks of pre-notice that you may or may not choose to notice and acknowledge it's still the same situation.

And the same rerun dilemma. What to do, how to protect yourself from being a victim of psychiatric abuses. How to get better in the most effective and quickest way possible so that you don't end up dead. It is a brutal illness that kills thousands yearly.

According to the *The Centers for Disease Control and Prevention* in 2013 (most current statistics available) it is estimated 41,149 persons in the U.S. took their own life. Some mental health professionals feel that is a low estimate, with many suicide deaths going unreported.

Quoted from *WebMD.com: Bipolar Disorder Health Center*:

"People with bipolar disorder are 10 times to 20 times

more likely to commit suicide than people without bipolar disorder. Tragically, 8% to 20% of people with bipolar disorder eventually lose their life to suicide."

Source: Rapid Cycling Bipolar

http://www.webmd.com/bipolar-disorder/guide/rapid-cycling-bipolar-disorder?page=2

Finding the way to the best end result with as low a risk and least harm done as possible; that's the challenge. It's no wonder bipolar persons are often very successful in business. Our souls have to be managed much like a national corporation, whether we like it or not.

Flying high and cutting deals: Is it this drug or that one that will work this time? Which one will have the least side effects and pose the least risk of causing me to cycle?

Collaborating with the most effective local professionals: Do I have to see a shrink and risk hospitalization (and my job, or any other current stability I may have successfully accomplished) or am I ok with the current plan and will try to ride out this downturn?

All the while constantly seeking better ways to do business, i.e. live your life while managing this illness. Electromagnetic fields have been used successfully in Canada, should I try it? Can I afford it? Is it cost-effective? Where is that risk analysis person I asked for? I have been waiting 15 minutes and have a doctor's appointment to get to.

When it really comes down to it I've been extremely fortunate. The hospitalizations I have had have been fairly brief, few and far in-between with the longest approximately two weeks. At the time of completing this book (in the makings for over 20 years) I am 49 years old and thankfully have not seen the inside of a mental ward in 24 years or so.

In addition, when I was hospitalized I was never mistreated. I was never abused or assaulted unlike many others who report horrendous abuse in institutional settings. If you are not familiar with the history of mental illness or some of the horror stories from years past and the sadistic doctors who ran the show rent the movie "Frances" starring Jessica Lange.

It is based on the true story of Frances Farmer, a brilliant woman and actress who was institutionalized for years and suffered tremendous abuse: repeated rapes, gang rapes from local soldiers (confirmed by staff), beatings, water torture, forced electroconvulsive therapy (ECT).

That she got a transorbital lobotomy which was gruesomely depicted in the film—a needle shoved into the eye socket with no anesthesia given to the patient—was denied by hospital staff, family and friends; it is assumed it was added to the film for effect.

Source: Shedding Light on Shadowland

http://jeffreykauffman.net/francesfarmer/sheddinglight.html

Yet the barbaric procedure was performed on over 300 patients at the hospital in the 1940s: Western State Hospital in Washington State.

Warning: The film is not for the faint-hearted. And anyone reading this book who does have some understanding of bipolar illness would most likely agree that just because it was not diagnosed and treated at that time, it is most likely what this incredibly talented and gifted woman suffered from.

She may have been given the diagnosis of Manic Depression but before the 1980s it would have been looked at more as a personality disorder, character flaws, lacking in self-control and discipline. Then treated with the 'why don't you just get over it' approach and if you don't, we are going to punish you because you are a bad person.

If I am understanding correctly from my brief research, it was not until 1980 that bipolar was used as a term in the official Diagnostic and Statistical Manual of Mental Disorders (DSM) and identified as a valid physical illness affected by chemical changes in the brain; a medical condition as opposed to a personality or character flaw that the patient had control over.

Quoted from *Healthline.com: History of Bipolar Disorder*:

"The term 'bipolar'—which means 'two poles' signifying the polar opposites of mania and depression—first appeared in the American Psychiatric Association's *Diagnostic and Statistical Manual of Mental Disorders* (DSM) in its third revision in 1980."

Source: Healthline.com - History of Bipolar Disorder

http://www.healthline.com/health/bipolar-disorder/history-bipolar

The abuse she endured at the hands of the psychiatric community in a forced five year incarceration was criminal. Her attending physicians should have been charged, convicted and jailed, even years later. And of course the soldiers as well.

I, on the other hand, was never tortured or abused when hospitalized. I was never held down and forced medication. I was never locked in solitary confinement or strapped to a bed for days on end. I was never physically or sexually assaulted.

I was also not given unwanted ECT therapy like many patients have had done—though at times my mental state made it seem like a very real threat. And at times it was a real threat, though as the saying goes: I dodged that bullet.

I remember a very frightening time of being strapped down in an acute care facility, ready to be transferred to a facility for a longer stay and begging to not have ECT—something I knew the facility participated in. That was true and real, the psych ward connected to the emergency room at Harborview Medical Center in Seattle, WA. where I was being evaluated.

On my way down but still pretty high, I was sure that was what they had in mind and my gurney along with the other drugged up co-patients beside me was lined up exactly for that purpose. I wasn't being transferred. I was being tricked. I was going to get the electrodes gooey-stuck to my temporal lobe with conductive gel and then jolted with electric currents.

They were preparing to bombard my cerebral cortex with volts of electricity to induce seizures, turn me into a temporary zombie and potentially cause long-term memory loss. Mechanical power charges that I knew were brain damaging, no matter what the psych establishment propaganda machine tried to promote. I could hear the zapping going on in the next room, I was sure of it.

Another time I flipped while living in a small waterfront community a few hours from Seattle. That was the time I took a fantasy trip into the jungle and became very psychotic in a very short amount of time. There was no preceding event to this manic episode (usually there is a clear ramp-up phase for me) except being in a new living situation and drinking something out of the fridge.

After being picked up by the cops and held for a few hours they transferred me to a crisis way station of sorts where I was evaluated by a psychiatrist. As usual, I was given antipsychotic or mood stabilizing medication and told I would be transferred again in a few hours.

Where did I end up? Western State Hospital, the same one depicted in the movie about Frances Farmer. I grew up in Seattle, did not know her story until years later (we had no history of mental illness in our immediate family until mine) but was very familiar with the lore surrounding the state mental institution not far away; everyone was.

What do you think I was thinking and feeling when I realized they were taking me there? The thoughts I could grab onto through the deluge of mind-altering drugs being administered were submerged in feelings of absolute terror. I would never leave, ever. They would drug me, force ECT, not listen to my wishes and create a mental nightmare I would never return from.

"I told you little one, we were waiting for your return, you think we are now going to let you go?"

What happened? I was admitted, had a young, sharp

attorney who handled the brief commitment hearing—let's call her 'angel'—and my stay was for the required 14 days. Came down on whatever antipsychotic or major tranquilizer I was given and managed to play a few competitive games of ping pong with Big Ben.

Another activity I remember is a mid-morning calisthenics class led by a sweet gal who had us standing on our tip toes, reaching up towards the sun. We all needed a little light.

And then what happens? Time's up. I left.

I liked Big Ben. A tall, lanky, late teen (early 20s?) who looked at me as I looked at him—on the inside (from within the walls of the funny farm) the same as one would on the outside. I'm sure he was as curious as to why I was in there as I was about him and the reasons why he had to be locked up.

Ben was a great distraction and so cute I couldn't resist calling out loudly "Big Ben!" when he would walk into the commons room; as if he were a sports star and I his number one fan. We were both clearing out of crisis mode, chemically responding to whatever major doses of psychotropic medications were being administered at the time.

Big Ben's time was up before mine (I think that is correct, it has been a while) so I got his address and promised to write. One of those intentions and follow throughs that reconnect a self to life. Five years or so his senior and taking on the caring big sister role I sent him a short note a few months later saying what a cool person I thought he was and to stay out of psych wards, I mean, trouble.

I didn't expect a reply back but if he had I would not have received it. Within the next three months or so later I would move out of the temporary apartment—moving on and moving ahead, trying to put as much distance between my re-stabilized self and the experience of being incarcerated as possible.

An experience that would be recreated in many forms from that time on—through travel abroad, relocation, changing jobs, friends, habits... whatever felt right or was forced upon myself in having to deal with the illness as well as post-traumatic stress from a mugging and sexual assault.

Moving became a salve to the soul and a very necessary escape in many senses of the word. An escape needed as much as the outpatient treatment and brief psychiatric follow-up visits that were asked of me by the community outreach program when re-entering society.

A couple visits and no more psychosis and that was the end of that. Life goes on, insurance is pricey, resources are scarce. I was fortunate to have the assessment that I was stable be correct and not have another experience of mania or major depression that resulted in hospitalization for years afterwards.

When you have a mental illness or have had an episode of mental incompetence such as a brief hospitalization and are a self-determined, independent person it can seem impossible to fit into society at all. The role that is imposed on you from that moment on is that of patient and subhuman.

You are supposed to subjugate yourself to others. To

those deemed more worthy and of value as members of society i.e. anyone who has not been labeled mentally ill. This includes of course the gatekeepers—psychiatrists and psychologists—as well as any other person in the world, with the possible exception of criminals and drug abusers. You've been placed into a societal niche whether you like it or not and had better stay there and behave or else.

Once hospitalized the threat—real or imagined—of another forced psychiatric stay can seem omnipresent. At least until enough time has passed and a level of competency attained such as a successful job, creative endeavor, relationship or other life-affirming event such as marriage or the birth of a child that has one once again feeling invincible, like the illness is gone.

You are well, even without the benefit of a cure. You are a human being again with enough distractions to forget the earlier incidences, for the time being.

Until another event occurs if one is so unfortunate yet for most persons with true bipolar illness highly likely. Then you are forced to re-enter the medical model of treatment; regurgitating for the millionth time your first episode 18 plus years earlier and all subsequent effects, treatments and possible causes hence since and what else have you done with your life?

"How are things?"

During one of these periods I'd had it with the reminiscing and of having to go over my history with professionals charging an average $100 per hour to sit and ask questions and listen. Isn't there such a thing called medical records? Aren't health professionals obligated if not mandated to review a patient's history of illness when accepting a patient for treatment?

It felt like mental torture after a time (or much unwanted use of brain cells at the very least) to be my own personal walking-talking medical USB and have to repeat traumatizing events over and over. Verbally repeat so that the professionals could sit on their lazy arses and pretend they are the latest and greatest addition to an already overlong course of years of treatment. When in actuality they had made their decision about me and how to proceed with treatment prior to even meeting me.

"And how about that new drug?"

Yes, I would have understandably been a bit bored yet sincerely trying to help at the same time as well if I was wearing their professionally trained shoes yet committing to a patient's care requires a bit of effort and willing, honest good intention; neither side of the couch is a cake walk.

Even worse, you have to process your life once again as a failure, a personal failure with or without the acknowledgement of a known mental illness thrown in. The years that I had fought to be well, to treat biological causes in addition to potential psychological contributing factors to my episodes of depression and mania had failed.

Your trust in yourself no matter how brilliant, composed, loveable, good-hearted or any other deserved, attributable quality is destroyed. How can you trust a self that has led you down a path of involuntary psychiatric hospitalization? A self that took away any sense of self-directedness you thought you had possessed or obtained?

Or worse still is the feeling of premonition that you are re-entering a void. The psychiatric void. They've got you now and there is no turning back. You thought you could spurn their help, assistance and domineering control? How silly. You thought you were well and a 'normal person'?

"Ha, ha again and welcome back, little one. You are in our clutches for real now, don't think you can escape."

Scary stuff, that void. Yet that fantasy picture isn't far from the truth when it comes to treatment modalities and living with Bipolar I Disorder.

When I was originally diagnosed in 1984 compliance was a primary goal of all forms of treatment with 'drug holidays'—a day the patients were allowed to skip a dose of their prescribed medications—one effort of many to encourage compliance with medical approaches to treatment. In the 20 plus years that followed little in that regard had changed.

The problem with this focus of treatment is that it rarely, if ever, works. And alas, I was to become one of its many statistical ready failures. You don't have to count them up.

CHAPTER 11

Bipolar Onset, Acknowledging Illness & Contributing Factors

In my case there were always thought to be possible underlying biological factors contributing to my symptoms, other than simply a brain gone off the tracks independently in and of itself. Once diagnosed as bipolar you don't get to say (or at least I haven't) that no, I'm really not. I have this or that illness, not bipolar... unless it was a true misdiagnosis by an incompetent or misinformed physician.

Or to say that you are cured. At this time there is no cure.

But that doesn't mean you do not have other medical issues that may be contributing to your bipolar states. Or that your actual bipolar illness did not come into existence i.e. the underlying genes giving expression, coming out of the woodwork of your DNA so to speak, to do their thing that happens to be f'ing with your brain cells and brain chemistry... because of outside factors that triggered its arrival.

"I'm here little one, now what are you going to do?"

And with that as a basic premise, how smart would it be to try and find those underlying factors and see if there are treatments available to either eliminate or control them. I've had some smart docs and have learned much from them. Now I am trying to share that learning and 'way of thinking about this illness' with you so that you can help yourself and try things or seek out appropriate medical care.

I know how frustrating it is to feel sick, be sick and feel there is no help available other than things you've tried that you do not want to do again. Like certain medications, like a visit to a looney bin—those kinds of things. For those with Bipolar I Disorder it may be next to impossible to avoid at least the major medication part during episodes. Some do well with maintenance doses of lithium and take it for life, feeling the side effects are worth suffering as the illness itself is worse.

I wish that was me but it isn't. I had to go off the drug in order to improve. I had to find other ways to be well.

For those with less severe forms of the illness like Bipolar II Disorder or Cyclothymic Disorder you may have excellent results in eliminating many of your symptoms by finding and treating underlying contributing factors. Hypomania is not a severe illness state and it could be a problem in your life due to diet (reactive hypoglycemia), side effects from meds, undiagnosed allergies, a need for better sleep habits and stress reduction, etc.

How to approach this issue from a biological angle? The first step (that your docs have most likely already done whether they shared it with you or not) is to analyze what happened at the onset of your illness. Did you take street drugs? Be honest. Were you on any new medications? Took over-the-counter meds?

Did you move to a new location? Remodel your home? Used pesticides or other toxic materials or were exposed to a high dose of them?

The way I look at onset is that of course it is the start of the illness (then from the date of onset you can track progression, remissions, etc.) but it is also the 'why' of it starting. That is what kept psychiatrists searching a bit for other undiagnosed illnesses in my case, in addition to treating the Bipolar I Disorder.

It's a lot easier to identify and treat those than it is to go the route Sexy 2 was and try the sledge hammer medication approach. Plus gives much better long-term results. All psychotropic medications are toxic and all have serious side effects. Have you ever heard of the 'serotonin syndrome'? No? Most likely your doctor has. That guy or gal writing the prescription for your medications.

"For more than 35 years psychiatrists have been aware of the serotonin syndrome—caused by use of multiple agents that increase levels of serotonin."

"The serotonin syndrome includes cognitive, autonomic nervous system, and somatic symptoms. Cognitive symptoms include: agitation, hypomania, headache, mental confusion, hallucinations, and coma. Autonomic symptoms include: shivering, sweating, fever, hypertension, nausea, and diarrhea. Somatic symptoms include: muscle twitching and tremor."

Source: <u>Amino Acid Therapy Q&A by David Gersten, M.D.</u>

The psychotropic medication prescribed to treat your bipolar illness can not only cause side effects, it can cause you to cycle or worsen whatever state you are in like my depression getting worse with lithium treatment.

The below information is from the article *Psychiatric Drug Facts – What Your Doctor May Not Know* on Peter Breggin, M.D.'s website. Dr. Breggin is a psychiatrist and court appointed scientific expert on cases involving psychiatric malpractice and liability for damages caused by psychotropic medications.

"Psychiatric drugs are more dangerous than you have ever imagined. If you haven't been prescribed one yet, you are among the lucky few. If you or a loved one are taking psychiatric drugs, there is hope; but you need to understand the dangers and how to minimize the risk."

"Antipsychotic drugs, including both older and newer ones, cause shrinkage (atrophy) of the brain in many human brain scan studies and in animal autopsy studies. The newer atypicals especially cause a well-documented metabolic syndrome including elevated blood sugar, diabetes, increased cholesterol, obesity and hypertension."

"They also produce dangerous cardiac arrhythmias and unexplained sudden death, and they significantly reduce longevity. In addition, they cause all the problems of the older drugs, such as Thorazine and Haldol, including tardive dyskinesia, a largely permanent and sometimes disabling and painful movement disorder caused by brain damage and biochemical disruptions."

Source: <u>Are All Psychiatric Drugs Too Unsafe To Take?</u>
http://www.breggin.com/index.php?option=com_content&task=view&id=3
16

In addition to the serious side effects outlined above for medications that may be prescribed to treat your bipolar illness, there are MANY substances that can affect brain chemicals that you may not be aware you have been exposed to (ingested or absorbed through the skin or airways).

You may not know you have had toxic exposures and also not be aware of the effects they could be having on your system which is affecting your bipolar illness i.e. your highs and lows.

And if these substances can adversely affect your brain and other organs, they can trigger the ONSET of bipolar or other illness. They don't create your genetic code that is the background—the operating system if you will—contained in the cells of your body but simply allow its expression i.e. the Crazyland theme wallpaper introduced in previous text. And who the heck wants to be crazy?

"Hang in there little one, there is always hope."

Or how about being exposed to a virus such as Epstein-Barr and having your system run down and your immune system not able to effectively keep viral numbers in check. This precipitates a chain reaction where the chemical changes caused by the viral illness begin a descent into depression and that triggers a first episode of bipolar illness you did not even know you had.

Until, like I did at age 19, you do normal things to treat symptoms and end up triggering the manic phase of the illness.

Other sufferers such as the talented news anchor, journalist and talk show host Jane Pauley have had similar experiences. They were being treated for depression (a horrible illness in and of itself) and given an antidepressant with a stimulant effect. The antidepressant causes chemical changes in the brain that then trigger a manic episode.

As an unfortunate end result they get hip (real fast) to the reality of their particular biochemical vulnerability. In treating the depression they learn they are bipolar.

"Hi, little one... what is your name?"

From what I have read of her story, for Jane the depression was from taking steroids to treat hives. She then had a few rounds of antidepressants with one eventually causing her to spiral into mania. My guess? It was in the tricyclic class of drug. Most psychiatrists will not prescribe an antidepressant for a Bipolar I patient without a major mood stabilizer taken also to prevent cycling into mania.

I remember reading an article about her in a magazine and being jealous that this lucky bipolar gal actually got to have a life before becoming ill. Not have her life (career, marriage, family) potentials halted at an early age due to the illness. She was diagnosed in her late 40s; lucky lady coming from the perspective of someone diagnosed in her late teens.

And she understood the basis of her illness plus didn't seem to have other major health issues. Me? Not so lucky.

Even though diagnosed with Manic Depression (what it was still called in the 1980s) I had fatigue and daytime drowsiness that started before I had a major depressive episode, not after. And it did not improve with treatment for depression, except one time with the tricyclic drug that then had to be stopped due to heart palpitations.

It was back to these more 'normal' illnesses such as thyroid disease and CFS/ME I went in search of trying to get better and stop feeling so sick and tired all the time. When I had my first manic episode I felt physically ill for days prior. I was nauseous, tired—like I had the flu but I didn't really have the flu.

And that was always included in my history. I had the lymph nodes in my neck felt on many occasions.

CHAPTER 12

Is Bipolar I Disorder More Severe Than Bipolar II Disorder?

The answer is yes. Bipolar I Disorder is a more severe form of this mental illness. It is the classic Manic Depression that has been around for ages. Bipolar II Disorder is a new psychiatric category created in 1994 with publication of the DSM-IV.

Here is a definition of Bipolar Type 1 quoted from the *John Hopkins Medical Center* website:

"People with Bipolar Type 1 experience mania consisting of distinct periods of persistently elevated, expansive or irritable mood. The mania may involve delusional ideas and impaired judgment. A manic episode is diagnosed if elevated mood occurs with three or more other symptoms for most of the day, nearly every day, for one week, or longer."

Source: Bipolar Type 1 or 2: How to Tell the Difference

http://www.johnshopkinshealthalerts.com/alerts/depression_anxiety/bipolar-disorder-types_6030-1.html

It does not mean that someone diagnosed with Bipolar II Disorder does not suffer much and possibly require treatment and medication to manage their illness. It simply means that the illness is a less severe form, with no mania present.

This is an important distinction to make. I have spent a little time participating in online bipolar support groups recently and there is a fair amount of confusion as to what the difference between the two diagnoses actually is, especially by BP-2 folks. Not only is there confusion, it seems there are some BP-2 sufferers who envy those who suffer from BP-1 or somehow feel inferior. It is like they are jealous BP-1 folks get all the attention and have all the fun. Or that their illness (and in extension themselves) is not as serious or important.

Of course not. Bipolar II Disorder can be very serious and require hospitalization for the depressive states, same as BP-1. Yet this would be an exception to the rule and not the norm. BP-2 usually does not lead to extreme mood states requiring inpatient care.

Much of how either illness will play out in the person's life depends simply on how responsive to available treatments the person is. It's a crap shoot of sorts and no one can predict a final outcome though the patient, physician, friends and family members are all hoping for the best. We all want to win at this game and thrive in our lives, not just survive.

BP-1 types on the other hand get clued in pretty quickly as to the severity of what they have been diagnosed with. It is difficult to not acknowledge going psychotic and having forced hospital stays. Not an easy thing to keep secret either.

On one lab visit getting a blood draw to check lithium levels before reporting back to Sexy 2 an old high school classmate was working in the area as a medical student. "Hi Molly, why are you in here?" Oh I see, checking lithium levels… hmmm, is someone bipolar?

Hot tip: If you have a need to maintain privacy about your mental illness move somewhere you did not spend a majority of your younger years and know a significant subset of the population. It is more than strange to be out walking around on a day pass during a hospital stay and run into someone you hadn't seen in years.

"Hi Molly, how are you, what have you been up to?" "Oh not much... I'm on my way back to the psych ward in a sec, room 204, how about you?" I could not get away from the person fast enough.

In all honesty, I would trade histories and brain patterns any day with a majority of those who have been diagnosed with BP-2. And also let them walk in my previous episodes shoes and see how they perceive the illness afterwards. I'll even go visit them in the psych ward. It is my guess they would be grateful it's not what they suffer from.

That is if they can actually survive an approximate four years of that hell without committing suicide or ending up placed in a long-term psychiatric care facility due to hypomania or a period of rapid cycling progressing into an actual manic state that does not respond to available treatments.

No cheating. And at least one Christmas must be spent destitute in a homeless shelter plus add in a bunch of intractable, pinching nerve pain that has you wanting to take a hammer and smash your hip to smithereens; anything to stop the pain. Survive that and my guess is the person will be thankful beyond belief they were not diagnosed with Bipolar I Disorder.

Bipolar Type 2 (BP-2) is defined by the *John Hopkins Medical Center* as follows:

"People with Bipolar Type 2 experience what's called hypomania, a mild to moderate level of mania that is generally a less destructive state than mania. Hypomania may feel good to the person who experiences it and may even be associated with good functioning and enhanced productivity. Impaired judgment is rare."

Source: Bipolar Type 1 or 2: How to Tell the Difference

http://www.johnshopkinshealthalerts.com/alerts/depression_anxiety/bipolar-disorder-types_6030-1.html

In short, Bipolar II Disorder typically does not require hospitalization, is more responsive to available medications and has a lower rate of permanent disability. As stated above, that does not mean a person with BP-2 does not have a difficult time in life dealing with mood swings, periods of depression or hypomania but that the emotional-biochemical states are most often not of the same magnitude as those experienced by a BP-1 sufferer.

Here is an excerpt from an excellent *Psychology Today* article on the subject: *Is Bipolar II Easier to Live with Than Bipolar I?*

"If you're unfortunate enough to live on the more unstable end of BP-I continuum, then life indeed can be rough. In this realm of the illness we see conditions that are highly unstable and treatment resistant."

"Traditional medication approaches are ineffective, relapse is frequent and symptom acuity is severe. Essentially these individuals are disabled by their BP-I disorder and they're often living on the margins of society."

"According to researchers Jamison and Goodwin (2007), this is the case for approximately 1/3 of those with BP. For these individuals, the bipolar illness is truly disabling"

Source: Bipolar You – The Young Adults Guide to Bipolar

http://www.psychologytoday.com/blog/bipolar-you/201210/is-bipolar-ii-easier-live-bipolar-i

Living on the margins of society, unresponsive to treatment, severe illness episodes... sounds very similar to my past life as a young adult living in the U.S. The article does not even include the issue of suicide. I almost successfully ended my life during that time; wanting to take myself out of the matrix of existence and put an end to the suffering.

A tendency towards depression is one thing Bipolar I Disorder and BP-2 do have in common. Both forms of the illness include the possibility of a serious depressive episode that may require hospitalization and may be unresponsive to treatment.

At present time I am stable for someone who has lived with Bipolar I Disorder for 30 years. Far from perfect and not high functioning unfortunately (I can only handle part-time work) but stable. I am not under the care of a psychiatrist, I am not taking any major doses of psychotropic medication and do not require treatment at this time.

Presently I am living life more like someone who has BP-2 (from the description given above) than someone suffering from BP-1 and have for years. A life possibly similar to someone who has been diagnosed with Bipolar II Disorder but of course not the same as. My Crazyland theme can go really berserk.

By comparison, the craziness experienced by BP-2 sufferers is much tamer and causes less disruption of the person's life.

When the various treatments I had during my twenties (described in the "*Things That Helped Me That May Help You or a Loved One*" chapter) helped to lessen the severe states of the illness I moved forward in life and did not require the same level of medical care i.e. had no major manic episodes that progressed to psychosis or suicidal depressions landing me a bed in a psych ward.

I was not stuck in survival mode and able to thrive. I worked, took excellent care of my son, socialized and enjoyed life for the most part.

Another way to look at it is that I got lucky. I've escaped long-term incarceration in the psych void even though I have a form of this illness that is debilitating and very difficult to treat successfully. I not only had to play doctor roulette for many years, I was constantly throwing the dice onto the table placing bets that this drug/vitamin/therapy would help or that treatment would be the one to give me a more stable, high-functioning existence.

It is a very difficult game to not only play, but to win.

There are some—I am in this camp—who feel that bipolar in general is currently being erroneously over-diagnosed. Not misdiagnosed as they've made-up new official categories for a whole new spectrum of bipolar (and widened the ages given the diagnosis i.e. children and the defenseless elderly) but erroneously.

Patients wrongfully labeled with the bipolar label with the primary reason an all-powerful pharmaceutical industry who wants to drug a larger portion of the population to increase profits. And psychiatrists (not all, but many) who play puppet to their demands to keep their insurance payments flowing in, BMW's painted the colors they prefer.

Those who used to be given the diagnosis of depression are now a new kind of bipolar. Instead of searching for more effective antidepressants or other treatments to help a sufferer recover and feel better the patient is forced to take on an additional burden of a new (unfounded) diagnosis and pressure to take a never-ending stream of harmful drugs.

I hear now of people on seven or more different psychotropic medications. Seven? More than one or two is insane unless absolutely necessary. Of course the need for many of them is to counteract the side effects of others rather than a dosage lowered or a medication discontinued when found to be ineffective or causing harm. It is medical malpractice.

Licensed physicians don't know how to read? Prescribe drugs without educating themselves about potentially harmful effects these medications may have on their patients?

That was not written to offend, but to inform. If you want to learn more, read *The Guardian* article *The Bipolar*

Explosion by British psychoanalyst Darian Leader. It outlines the new categories of bipolar appearing in connection to an expiring drug patent and need to market a new class of antipsychotic medications.

Source: The Bipolar Explosion

http://www.theguardian.com/commentisfree/2012/jun/20/bipolar-explosion-psychiatry-mental-health

Sound fishy? It is and is also—in my humble opinion—heinous. If you understood the damage psychotropic medications can cause and how truly difficult and life-altering the illness of Manic Depression is you would understand my strong feelings on the matter.

We now have 'bipolar children'. What? You mean super bright, energetic beings of light with limitless potential who have come into this world to live, learn and love and what do we do? Label and then force harmful toxic substances into their growing, vulnerable bodies.

What about children who are being abused (incest, over-strict authoritarian parenting negatively affecting a sensitive child, emotional neglect from a drug addicted parent, physical abuse) and parents seeking a psychiatric diagnosis to label the child the 'problem' and absolve themselves from responsibility?

Those are complicated issues but incredibly important to be aware of and publicly discuss. Drugging children with brain damaging medications is not acceptable psychiatric or medical care; it is abuse.

CHAPTER 13

Major Depression is Hell

Depression is as important a topic to write about as is the fact we need better treatments for depression. As mentioned in the previous chapter, many people are suffering—horribly—from severe depression and then mislabeled 'bipolar' because they are not being treated successfully.

Just because your depression is not being treated successfully does not mean you have bipolar disorder. And you should thank your lucky stars for that.

My depressive phases of my bipolar illness have been horrific. Best word I can come up with but let me try to elaborate with help from my writing companion Google. A few synonyms for the word 'horrific' according to *Oxford Dictionaries.com* are: dreadful, horrendous, frightful, fearful, awful, terrible, atrocious, harrowing, unspeakable, monstrous, ghastly and nightmarish. I concur with all of the above.

Heinous was also included in the list but I've already used that term to describe the licensed professionals who are mislabeling depressed individuals bipolar. Mislabeling with the primary purpose of then being able to drug to infinity these suffering people with brain disabling antipsychotic meds. Drugging while ignoring the dangerous side effects these medications have. So we will let that one stand as is.

The depressive phase of BP-1 is called Major Depression or a 'major depressive episode'. Major Depressive Disorder is a separate classification of mood disorder than bipolar and is also referred to as 'clinical depression' or 'unipolar depression'.

Some people with bipolar illness experience many depressive episodes during their lifetime. Others may only have one incidence of Major Depression during the course of their illness; lucky ducks. The same goes for elevated moods progressing to mania with some sufferers having many episodes of mania while others experience only one manic episode.

The illness Major Depressive Disorder is much more common than the illness Manic Depression. The below is quoted from the *Stanford School of Medicine Depression Research Clinic*:

"Major Depression, also known as clinical or unipolar depression, is one of the most common mental illnesses. Over 9 million American adults suffer from clinical depression each year."

"Major Depression is more than a temporary state of feeling sad; rather, it is a persistent state that can significantly impair an individual's thoughts, behavior, daily activities, and physical health."

Source: What is Depression?

Those who have never experienced serious depression may wonder why those who have are such big, whiny babies. Just get over it already and on with your life, they may think. We all have difficulties at times and experience loss, disappointment that makes us feel sad. Why can't you deal with it like other normal people do?

Because those with Manic Depression experiencing a major depressive episode or those who have been diagnosed with Major Depressive Disorder are not like normal people.

They—same as me when overtaken by this mood state—can't get over it on their own. It doesn't go away and does not get better. Maybe it will eventually but when it has a stranglehold over your life you cannot fathom having to survive another day feeling so dreadfully awful. Feeling worse than you ever imagined possible and barely being able to move much less think clearly. You have lost all hope of ever feeling better again. The depression has become an illness needing some form of outside assistance. It is not just a temporary period of sadness or heightened anxiety.

You are sick.

This is when thoughts of suicide invading your brain won't relent. They are in it for the long haul and just keep getting stronger. Try and stop us, they say. They get louder and more persistent, pushing you to think of doing things you would never think of or consider doing if not in the depressive state. Ending your life and the suffering you are experiencing becomes an obsession. The only issues of importance are how and when and will I have enough courage to go through with it.

At these times I never realized I could be so determined, so persistent and so forceful in trying to force myself to do something i.e. commit suicide. I never dreamed I would ever even consider attempting suicide. Where have these thoughts and feelings come from? Is this really me, who I am? Am I this horrible of a human being?

Once I sat for an hour with a razor blade held at my neck. No more calls to the Suicide Prevention Center this time. I was going to do it. And not the wimpy female way which would land me in a psych ward. I wasn't looking for attention, I wanted to die. Use my deft fingers to feel for that major artery in my neck. Press the lethal blade into the skin... a little more pressure. One little cut and that carotid artery has got to start spurting and give me a speedy death; I will bleed out quickly, right?

Obviously I never went through with it but that is how bad it got a few times.

This is when states of existence outside of the depressive state are not present. You are withering away in that black hole out of the mainstream and you have had enough of being left out of the good times. You are through with having to have to push through day after day only to feel worse regardless of your efforts to feel better. No more of this, you say. I don't deserve to suffer. I deserve to be able to die and put an end to this suffering.

The depression has progressed into Major Depression and has become an illness needing intervention.

This is when a rapid cycling person like I have been at times during my life may switch into mania. You think maybe that would be a welcome change, right? You think that moving into a manic state would be fun, just what a depressed person needs to pull them out of their rut. Goodbye depression, hello good times.

All us BP-1 sufferers appreciate your kind thoughts and you rooting for us. We are thankful for your kind sympathy and wanting to see an end to our suffering and for us to feel more like you do. You are more of what the world needs.

Unfortunately, bouncing from wanting to die to having fun is not what usually happens. Good times are nothing close to what a true manic episode is. Mania is unstable, turbulent energy and out of control behavior. You feel restless and out of sorts. Or you are feeling too good to be true. This is fantastic!

Feelings of feeling great that often don't last long. Then comes the crash and burn. Then the wondering what the heck happened. And for those like me who can go from being manic to being psychotic pretty quickly... why the heck am I strapped to this hospital gurney? Why am I here and where are they taking me?

What I am trying to describe is how different the severe depression of Manic Depression—now called Bipolar 1 Disorder—is from the severe depression of Major Depressive Disorder. They have similar characteristics but require very different forms of treatment. Once you have been manic your care providers have to prevent the switch to mania when trying to save your life during a depressive phase.

That is what they are doing, trying to save your life. And what choices do they have at their disposal for treating you? You've already been in therapy most likely and your support system is worn out. What's next?

Drugs, lots of drugs. First attempts. Then more drugs. Second attempts. Treatment of co-existing illnesses if can be identified and the medical professional is astute enough to search for any, mainly as every other effort to help you has failed. Third attempts. New doctor and more diagnostic tests, maybe a brain scan. Still depressed and suicidal? Shock your brain and self into submission—a new altered state—try to at least with brain damaging ECT.

Not dead yet? Let's see... what else can we pull out of our hats? This is where we are at today in the treatment of depression. Still trying to pull the rabbit out of the hat and—surprise— a person suffering from depression is feeling better. Thank you sweet Jesus and hallelujah. Everyone is happy. It is a beautiful thing. Life goes on.

For many life does not go on, they end up dead. Treatment only causes worsening of symptoms. Suicidal ideation progresses into more active and aggressive suicide attempts that may be successful. Or worse, the prescribed psychotropic medication prompts uncharacteristic violent or criminal behavior in some individuals leading them to harm others.

Someone who has an inclination towards violence possibly gets triggered into action with the chemical reactions in their brain caused by their ingesting medication. Not street drugs but legal drugs prescribed by a physician or psychiatrist. They were being compliant with treatment and given the reward of being hospitalized, put in jail or shoveled into an early grave.

The below information is from the article: *Nearly Every Mass Shooting in the Last 20 Years Shares One Thing in Common.*

"In nearly every mass shooting in the United States in the last twenty years the perpetrator was either actively taking psychotropic medication or had been in the immediate past before they committed their crimes."

Source: WorldTruth.tv

http://www.sott.net/article/279716-Nearly-every-mass-shooting-in-the-last-20-years-shares-one-thing-in-common-and-it-isnt-weapons

Disturbing? It is beyond disturbing. The article lists details of the mass shootings as well as many suicides by teenagers that happened after they began taking psych meds. The main offenders? Antidepressant medications such as Prozac, Zoloft and Paxil.

Every human being on the planet has to ask why teenagers are still being prescribed these medications. And even more importantly demand to know why we do not have better treatments for depression. Why not? Scientists are stupid? Billionaire drug manufacturers can't fund more studies and report honestly and accurately about the results? The FDA is incapable of providing oversight?

With the information above plus numerous other studies that verify and illustrate the danger and long-term damaging health effects of these medications, why do doctors routinely hand out prescriptions for them? Why are they not banned from being prescribed to those under the age of 18 at minimum and long-term use discouraged?

The reason is they are the primary white, fluffy ploy we have to pull out of the hat when someone is suffering from severe depression and medical intervention is necessary. That is the identifiable problem. The solution is more treatment options and physicians willing to do more than just give out psychotropic medications like they are candy. We need more doctors like 'B for Brilliant' and The Dude who are up next.

More persons suffering from Major Depression or a depressive episode of Manic Depression should be given a range of treatment options to help them try to get well, feel better and stay well. Not just a prescription for an antidepressant or antipsychotic medication and bi-weekly chat sessions.

When in crisis, maybe if absolutely necessary. When dealing with an intermittently reoccurring, chronic medical condition such as Manic Depression or Major Depressive Disorder, no. Chronic illness will most likely be made worse with long-term use of toxic medications, not better. If at all possible, it should be avoided.

The below is quoted from *HelpGuide.org – Depression Medication*:

"A major National Institute of Mental Health study showed that fewer than 50 percent of people become symptom-free on antidepressants, even after trying two different medications. Furthermore, many who do respond to medication soon slip back into depression, despite sticking with drug treatment."

"Other studies show that the benefits of depression medication have been exaggerated, with some researchers concluding that—when it comes to mild to moderate depression—antidepressants are only slightly more effective than placebos."

Source: <u>What You Need to Know About Medications for Depression</u>

http://www.helpguide.org/articles/depression/antidepressants-depression-medication.htm

Patients and their families need more education about things they can do on their own and more access to alternative treatments like I have had—after an initial crisis has passed. Long-term use of psychotropic medications (antidepressants, antipsychotics, mood stabilizers) should be rare, not commonplace. Let me illustrate further by sharing with you a few of the many alternative treatment options available; ones that have helped me.

CHAPTER 14

Things That Helped Me That May Help You or a Loved One

feeding into that impulse only makes things worse and prolongs the suffering. I read during one of these times something on a website a crisis intervention counselor had written. I cannot remember it word for word but it was basically that when someone gets to the point where they are thinking of harming themselves it is a sign that "the pain has temporarily exceeded their ability to cope".

Emphasis on temporary; things always change, this too will pass. Your coping skills will return.

Treating an underlying hypothyroid issue and unknown chemical sensitivities (detoxing from exposures), taking vitamin and mineral supplements, probiotics, salmon oil (large doses to almost puking), removing mercury fillings and diet changes (no more sugar) helped much in healing and preventing additional manic and severe depressive episodes. Not cure, but helped.

During my search to get well after operation overload on lithium failed I read a ton about causes of chronic fatigue. You can go bonkers trying out things that may or may not help and that is not something we want to encourage here (grin). But some of these issues may be an underlying factor in your illness as they were in mine and things that have helped me help you or a loved one.

Not all, but some.

And get ready for a bunch of fails and to be able to deal with it. None of these are a quick fix, none are going to transport you back to your 'pre-bipolar diagnosis and illness' state. But some may help you improve your health and to feel better. With that goal in mind I am happy to share what I have learned.

Most important is learning about the effects toxic exposures can have on your general health and how avoiding them (pesticides, formaldehyde saturated building materials, chemicals in new furniture, natural gas, toxic molds, etc.) can go a long way in lessening the symptoms and severity of any illness, including bipolar.

How did I learn much of this? Through the good fortune of getting to receive care from yet another highly skilled doc; we will call him Dr. B for Brilliant as that is what he is. Dr. B is an environmental medicine specialist and listened to my story and onset of illness with a new ear and different medical framework with which to try and find clues as to what was causing my symptoms. Or at least some of them.

He picked up on some key points that a psychiatrist will not pick up or focus on. Clues such as environmental triggers and toxins and in my case there were plenty. Pesticides were sprayed in the kitchen of our apartment in San Francisco every two weeks to keep cockroaches at bay. I had my clothes hanging on a store clothing rack (thought it was cool and the room had no closet) and we bombed the place for fleas, including all my clothing.

I got real busy with a project (surprise, surprise) of stripping the wood floors (toxic chemicals and no protection) and then refinishing them. The smells got me a little high, no bother. Sort of lifted me out of the mood I was in, gave a different feel, nothing wrong there.

Dr. B suggested that these exposures were a part of the puzzle of why I had an increase of fatigue and 'sleepy to the point of almost passing out' drowsiness in the afternoons. We went into detox mode and I read yet another ton of medical literature on how these exposures can impact health.

I did saunas, large doses of Vitamin C intravenously (to decrease viral levels and give my body a chance to get back doing that work on its own), basic vitamin and mineral supplementation, had mercury removed from teeth and to top it off, did live cell therapy at a clinic in Mexico. Again, to get my system to stop sloughing off and back on the program of functioning like a normal system should.

Sheesh, who the heck did it think it was anyways?

And I learned my triggers. Formaldehyde and exposure to natural gas will make me feel sick and get depressed very quickly. Same with Lysol and Windex cleaning products; it is like a virus is being activated. I get prickly chills, pain issues triggered, drowsy. The chills and worsening of symptoms will go away if I end the exposure (leave the room, get fresh air). That is not what would happen with an actual viral infection.

I did well with work after getting better and finishing college but when a company I was working at moved into a brand new office building, after a few months I knew I was starting to re-sensitize and would become more ill if I stayed in that environment. I hung in there as long as I could then it was time to leave.

I have done some regular medical stuff too such as taking a low dose of Prozac at times. But I was being treated by a general practice physician, not a psychiatrist. I was not only living out of the country at the time (Mexico) and did not have access to that type of care, I didn't want it.

I didn't want to have to recount my history for the zillionth time, demoralize myself more than I already felt demoralized. I just wanted to be treated as a person who was having a hard time and see what the doctor would recommend. I had an infected tooth and pain for many months as could not afford a root canal, part of what triggered the episode.

He was very kind and spoke English; that was a plus! I did share that I was bipolar but he simply expressed concern, not fear as though I was some crazy person whom he could not help and we decided together it would be ok to take a very low dose of Prozac. A low dose to try and lift me up out of the state I was in without triggering a mood switch.

I got lucky, it worked.

I was prescribed the lowest dose available and at the start think I even broke up the pill so it was even a lower amount of the drug. I knew what I was taking upon waking every morning would function more like a mild tranquilizer than antidepressant as the amount was not really enough to alter my brain chemicals much. It would have a slight effect on how I felt and hopefully help me slowly regain my ability to cope but most likely not trigger hypomania.

Important note: As of now, in 2016, I would never take Prozac - or any psychiatric medication - ever again unless somehow forced to (manic psychosis triggered). I did not understand the placebo effect of antidepresant medication before, now I do.

Source: <u>Understanding the Placebo Effect of Antidepressants</u>

http://www.bipolar1survivor.com/placebo-effect-antidepressants/

Less drug equals less effect on brain chemical levels means less chance of affecting other levels of brain chemicals that you are not trying to mess with, such as what happens with a switch from depression or a normal state to mania in a BP-1 person.

This type of treatment would have been hard to get in the U.S. as all you have to say is you are bipolar and automatically large doses of meds will be assumed to be the treatment of choice of whatever state you are in. If it is mild to moderate, at least in my case, I would never be at the doctor's office in the first place. So if I am complaining and seeking care it is significant, potentially serious, and the docs will pick up on that pretty quickly. Those folks aren't exactly mental lightweights.

It was a huge victory to seek care like a regular person (not a psychiatric patient), try something that would not be a big deal for them but was definitely unconventional for someone with my history and have it work. I used the same approach a couple of times later, even experimented with the low dose as a PMS cure but always after about two months the switch would start to a hypomanic state and I would have to stop taking it.

Since it has a long half-life I tried taking it day on, day off but that didn't work either. Even though I knew this was risky as it could prompt mood cycling I was sick of the cycling and willing to give it a try. I wanted out of the rat race going on inside my brain.

You do not win bipolar cellular control freaks but can we call a truce? Meet somewhere in the middle, find common ground and get on with our lives. How about live a productive life? That's an awesome goal to have.

Sharing this information is a part of accomplishing what this book is about i.e. to give an accurate depiction of what living with this illness is really like. And to help others who are suffering or who have a loved one who has been diagnosed as bipolar understand the dynamics of the illness while offering suggestions of things that may help.

Things you can do that may lessen the misery it causes.

CHAPTER 15

Treatments & Self Help Protocols

The treatments and self-help protocols I have done during these past two decades are described below to the best of my ability. I am not a licensed health care provider. I am just a layperson sharing information about living with Bipolar I Disorder and a few things I have discovered that helped reduce the intensity and occurrence of its severe states; at least for me.

I am hoping this information helps you or a loved one also. Some require working with a doctor, others you can do on your own. Try what feels right to you.

Please do not get your hopes up for or expect anything to be a miracle cure. There is no cure at this time but there are many things you can do that may help moderate your mood swings and help you balance your brain chemistry better. Help you feel better and move forward in life. Help you to thrive as opposed to just survive.

It is very important to note that anything new you try, even if it is only new foods added to your diet, can have an effect on medications you take. Be sure to take this into account and consult with your physician as needed.

1. Low Dose of Prozac

Taking the lowest dose of Prozac to pull out of a serious depression (living in Mexico, regular doctor) while not triggering a switch to mania helped much on a few occasions. But every time I had to go off the med after around two months as started to feel myself go through the physical change preceding a switch for me.

When I am starting to become hypomanic with a full-blown manic episode just up ahead around the next corner I begin to feel sick with some feelings of anxiety yet dull inside; like a calm before an impending storm.

I was prescribed Prozac to treat serious depression years prior but it was yet another fail. The reason? They prescribed too high a dose, and I did not understand my sensitivities to chemicals at the time. Same reason Sexy 2 was not successful in treating me.

Important note: As of today, 2016, I would not take Prozac or any psychiatric medication ever again. I now understand that they are not treating any identifiable chemical imbalance in a person's brain. I already know the harm they can cause.

Learn more here: *Would I ever take Prozac Again?*

Source: www.bipolar1survivor.com

http://www.bipolar1survivor.com/would-i-ever-take-prozac-again/

2. Thyroid Hormone

I haven't mentioned Dr. D ("The Dude") yet but will now. He is a specialist in bipolar disorder (or at least was, most likely is retired by now) at the University of Washington Medical School and my Dad paid a pretty penny ($400) for me to have a hour consult with him. He was also my attending physician during a hospital stay.

Dr. D. helped me greatly by prescribing a low dose of thyroid hormone, even though my blood levels were in the low normal range. It pulled me out of a severe depression and ended suicidal thoughts and feelings. It worked when the psychotropic meds weren't and is not a toxic drug.

This was not a common treatment approach at the time but just beginning to be studied. A research article published in *Psychiatry Online* in 2006 stated:

"A mounting scientific database documents the increased prevalence of medical comorbidity among persons with a mood disorder. For example, subclinical hypothyroidism is associated with recurrent depression, longer disease duration, more frequent affective episodes, repetitive nonlethal suicidal behaviors, and a higher body mass index."

Source: Medical Comorbidity in Bipolar Disorder: Implications for Functional Outcomes and Health Services Utilization

http://psychiatryonline.org/doi/full/10.1176/ps.2006.57.8.1140

I was one of those patients with a functional outcome

and who most likely had a coexisting medical condition of subclinical hypothyroidism – a mild form of hypothyroidism. I've taken a low dose of the thyroid medication Synthroid for twenty-four years with positive results and no problems. Unlike every other medication I was given to treat my bipolar illness i.e. all had distressing or dangerous side effects.

Synthroid can cause side effects (including put you into a hyperthyroid state) and you do need to make sure the dosage is correct. You have to have your blood levels checked after you start the med which any competent physician will do.

It took a couple of months to start to have an effect and for me to realize it was really helping but Synthroid made the daytime drowsiness I had been complaining about for years go away. Go away completely as in no more wanting to fall asleep during the day.

As the depression lifted the fatigue lessened but never went completely away and at times is debilitating. Sometimes I feel I've spent half my adult life resting. I have some type of affecting illness whether it is CFS/ME, Relapse-remitting Multiple Sclerosis (RRMS), worsening of fibromyalgia or other.

If I hadn't been mugged and sexually assaulted during those years (my mid-20s) I probably would have been higher functioning and moving forward in life sooner than I did.

If I go off of the hormone I won't notice any significant change for a week or month or longer (depending on what mood state I am in chemically). But then slowly those daytime drowsiness and increase in fatigue symptoms will start to resurface and can trigger a depressive state. Going back on a low dose of Synthroid gets them under control again.

It also helps stabilize my moods, accomplishing the baseline level of stability that lithium gives some people but did not work for me.

This is an avenue of care I have a renewed interest in. I have felt myself decline a little the past few years (ages 45-49) and have learned much more about thyroid issues and treatments. I wanted to be tested for 'free T3' levels during my most recent medical exam but the doc would not order the test. She would only test my T4 levels, as is common in our today's world of 'drug company dictated medical care'.

Synthroid is synthetic T4. Your T4 levels do not show how much of the more bioavailable form of thyroid hormone—T3—is circulating in your bloodstream. Your body makes more T4 but then converts much of it into T3. A few more steps and T3 becomes 'free T3' and it is free T3 in the tissues that is doing most of the good stuff at the metabolic level.

Testing free T3 levels is important, though the manufacturers of Synthroid would not want you to know that or your doctor to follow that protocol. If they are low you may want to try desiccated thyroid brands that are made from the actual gland and contain both T4 and T3. Natural Thyroid (NT) brands manufactured in the U.S. are Armour, NP Thyroid and Nature-throid.

How this may or may not help your bipolar illness I of course have no idea but it is something to think about, especially if fatigue or daytime drowsiness is a major symptom. Also, lithium can cause thyroid problems or make existing ones worse. Thyroid issues are a great topic for anyone to learn more about, but especially those with bipolar illness.

3. Avoid Toxic Exposures and Allergens

Most will not think of this unless they have done all the crazy alternative treatments I have, but it works. The basic concept to understand is that if you have become ill, something (or a few or many things) caused the illness whether they can be identified or not. The illness itself is the end result.

So put some effort into searching for those causes, to see if treatments are available that will help you eliminate or reduce their effects. Bipolar is an illness that affects levels of chemicals in the brain which in turn affect mood states. There are an endless number of factors to explore.

Beyond the obvious (B12 deficiency, anemia, thyroid issues, a tumor) you may also want to think of things in your environment that may be toxic or simply toxic to you, put you in an 'overload' state and cause symptoms such as gas heat, outgassing of new carpet or paint, a moldy basement, etc. Things that can be easily avoided.

And this also applies to triggers. Triggers are those

things that get a depression or wind-up phase going, set those train wheels on the track. When you drink milk or eat sugar how do you feel afterwards? After a day shopping (and getting an overload of chemical exposures) do you feel energized, almost hypomanic? Depressed? Does perfume give you a headache?

How about that new dryer sheet you do not need to put in your dryer. While taking your clothes out do you get nauseous? Irritable or anxious?

The best thing to do to pursue this line of thinking is simply to get online and start reading about environmental illness, chemical sensitivities, food allergies, etc. Focus on eliminating the things that unnecessarily add stress to your system. Protect your family by making your home a non-toxic, safe haven from the industrialized, polluted world we live in.

If you talk with your doctor about mold, allergies or noxious chemicals possibly contributing to your mood states and they poo poo the idea, giving you that 'you may actually be insane, not just bipolar' look... glance back at them sternly. Then remind him or her how their most holiest of holy professions used to routinely surgically remove the thymus gland as a treatment for cancer.

That is, until they discovered it was (is) the master gland of the immune system that controls most of its functions. Oops.

Just because they have no training in the field of environmental medicine or knowledge of how even minute exposures to harmful substances can impact health it does not mean you have to be ignorant to this reality as well.

If you have severe mood states and are unresponsive or over-responsive to psychotropic medications (substances that are non-natural and can be toxic) you may be sensitive to chemicals and benefit from reducing exposures and going through a period of detox.

This is not something to stress yourself out over or to get paranoid about. Chances are you are NOT chemically sensitive. Let's make sure you stay that way and do not unknowingly overwhelm your system with substances that could be easily avoided; exposures to toxins that would negatively impact your health and potentially worsen your bipolar illness and mood states.

The below quotes are from an *American Journal of Public Health* article:

"A report published by the National Academy of Sciences in 1981 said that 15% of the American population could have a heightened sensitivity to chemicals."

"A more recent random population study by the California Department of Health Services (CDHS) indicated a hypersensitivity prevalence of 15.9% in Californians surveyed."

Source: Prevalence of Multiple Chemical Sensitivities
http://www.ncbi.nlm.nih.gov/pmc/articles/PMC1448331/

Partly why I moved to Mexico years ago for an extended stay when my son was just 6 years old was I knew the hot weather, days at the beach and all-around less stressful style of living (that I could afford) would support continued detox of my system. Instead of adding new exposures such as working nine to five in a climate controlled office building would.

I was concerned about potential harm to my son—then a high energy, active toddler—as well. I was worried about the effects of being stuck on a freeway daily for hours (two or more was usual for our commute), inhaling exhaust fumes while strapped in his child safety seat. I did not want him to develop illness issues like Mom had experienced.

A website with easy to understand information about chemical sensitivity such as what it is, possible symptoms it may cause and what you can do to help your body heal is: Multiple Chemical Sensitivity.org.

http://www.multiplechemicalsensitivity.org/

4. Light Exercise Daily

I say daily but of course that does not happen. There are days when I am too fatigued, in pain or simply have too much on my plate to fit in any exercise as it would push me over the edge and cause more fatigue and pain (aggravate symptoms of CFS/ME or fibromyalgia). Yet most days I do get something in even if it is only a 15 minute walk, even if I do not feel like doing it. That is victorious for someone with my history. And something I have control over; the illness I do not.

If I ever get revved up to do a bunch of stuff I know to not do it all, try not to do too much. I realize that it is simply my brain starting to rev up. I may not have control over the wheels starting to churn within my cells but I do have control over my actions for the most part.

Sticking to a schedule of moderate, low impact exercise (take a walk, swim, gentle stretching and calisthenics, bike ride) as I am able and focusing on keeping calm can help my brain—and my self—get a grip.

When I was younger and able to handle aerobic exercise, I would try to work out as I could (swim, jog, play soccer) as I knew I would feel better after. I knew it would improve my mood or at least help keep my weight down and that would make me feel better. No one wants to look or feel unattractive.

Being a bit vain is an advantage to surviving this illness.

I tried yoga for relaxation and improved mood health but found it overwhelmingly boring in practice. I loved learning its history and about Eastern religions, with its mystics and yogis plus the cute outfits you got to wear to class. But my diligent efforts to stretch, relax, stretch some more to eventually reach nirvana only led to me feeling frustrated; it did not make me feel better.

What helps me feel better is to move... to get out and walk, breathe fresh air, let my mind wander as my feet advance one step in front of the other.

5. Sleep and Rest

Sleep is the biggie here as anyone with bipolar illness knows or hopefully has at least been told by their doctor or therapist how important it is. It is important to our well-being and to managing mood states, more so than for normal folks. And getting quality sleep is critical for all of us homo sapiens.

Lack of sleep, staying up all night, feeding into impulses to get riled up instead of chilling yourself the heck out (big one for me) can all trigger hypomanic and manic states. You have to tell your brain and body that YOU are in control, not that psychedelic print pattern it is waving on the horizon of your neurons. Take it off now you say, today is NOT going to be a Crazyland day! And then take a nap and possibly some melatonin (natural sleep aid) at night before bed to help you sleep.

You need deep sleep to shut down the operating system of your brain cells and force them into reset mode so you wake up refreshed; not just light sleep which may slow it down a bit while still up and running.

And download that Crazyland theme wallpaper to a flash drive, stick it in a drawer and keep it there until you choose to put it back up (what normal folks get to do) or your brain does without your consent (what happens to bipolar folks).

I write more about sleep and how it is connected to bipolar on my Bipolar 1 Survivor blog.

http://www.bipolar1survivor.com

6. Sunshine

Sunshine is an easy one to understand and becoming more understood in importance due to the high numbers of people diagnosed with Vitamin D deficiency as well as its effect on serotonin levels and the illness Seasonal Affective Disorder (SAD).

SAD can be a large contributing factor in some bipolar patient's illness. The depressive phase may be triggered during cold, light-less winter months and the hypomanic or manic phase occurring during the spring and summer due to the abundant amount of sunshine and extended hours of daylight. The change from one weather pattern to the other may affect a chemical switch in the brain from one mood state to the other.

The below is quoted from a *Current Psychiatry.com* article:

"Seasonal affective disorder (SAD) is an umbrella term for mood disorders that follow a seasonal pattern of recurrence. Bipolar I disorder (BD I) or bipolar II disorder (BD II) with seasonal pattern (BD SP) is the DSM-IV-TR diagnosis for persons with depressive episodes in the fall or winter and mania (BD I) or hypomania (BD II) in spring or summer."

Source: Is Seasonal Affective Disorder a Bipolar Variant?
http://www.ncbi.nlm.nih.gov/pmc/articles/PMC2874241/

My severe period of illness (rapid cycling, hospitalizations) was while I was living in Seattle, WA. That rainy, dreary, cloudy place that promoters (and avid gardeners) like to say has a 'Mediterranean climate'. Oh bite me, I offer in reply. Only 71 days of partial sunshine on average a year (300 plus cloudy days) does not remind me of our time living on the southern coast of Spain. I taught English a couple of months, my then 4 year old son tagged along and we spent many days at the beach.

I loved the climate and can promise you it bears little in resemblance to weather patterns in Seattle.

Snarky joking aside, it is a very cool city and great place to live if you are not bipolar with a tendency towards dreary weather-induced depression. I personally feel much better and have fewer depressive episodes when living in a sunny climate; a form of nature therapy that is free.

7. Eliminating Sugar from Diet and Candida

Since the drowsiness hit in the afternoons I was tested for blood sugar issues; all fine. But when learning about Candida overgrowth in the body (good microorganisms vs bad microorganisms colon wars) and how that can cause low moods and other symptoms and all the sugar I was ingesting without even realizing it I decided to try and eliminate sugar from my diet.

I was tested for overgrowth of Candida (a type of fungus) in my gut using a fecal sample. The doctor greeted me on the visit scheduled to discuss the results with a hearty, "Congratulations". I sat in the office chair looking a bit perplexed as to what could be cause for celebration and then he continued. He went on to inform me I had the highest level of Candida in my gut the test had ever registered.

Clearly this was a problem I needed to address, and most likely a strong contributor to my poor health issues.

At the time I had constant vaginal yeast infections with smelly, disgusting discharge and itchy to the point I would scratch myself sore. I had lovely anal itching as well. Over-the-counter creams made it yuckier with burning pain accompanying the itch. It would then improve for a short time but always returned.

After the test results I was given a prescription for an antifungal medication, told to take an acidophilus supplement plus avoid foods that contained yeast. No more beer, wine, bread, cheese, pickles, creamy salad dressings, etc. or foods that promote yeast overgrowth such as anything with processed sugar; basically all my favorite foods at the time. What fun.

In addition, when I splurged on something sweet I would get shaky and need to eat protein afterwards. I just finally got to the point where I said I have to stop eating this stuff and see how I feel. It was tough at first as I had an emotional as well as physical addiction to sugary goodness in foods but helped much.

No more hypoglycemic attacks, felt better all around and helps keep weight down.

At some point someone told me about medicinal uses of Boric acid powder and how it would kill the vaginal yeast.

After quite a few applications (tampon rolled in the white powder, inserted then taken out a few hours later removing a bunch of greenish-yellowish gunk) the yeast infections finally abated and the microflora of my private parts have remained blessedly in balance for the most part ever since.

I wanted to nominate them for a National Academy of Science award.

8. Gamma Globulin and Shark Cells

That subheading reads like an introduction to a new type of haunted house set-up to spook young children on Halloween but are actually two additional treatments I had. Both therapies are genius in theory and meant to help a compromised immune system kick back into gear and get up and running efficiently.

Yep, you guessed it, Dr. B strikes again.

Gamma globulin (also called immunoglobulin) is made from human blood plasma and contains a concentrated amount of antibodies—the good stuff that fights infectious agents in your body i.e. those vile organisms that are trying to take over the controls in your cells and make you sick. I received shots before I went off traveling to Asia many years ago.

I was very concerned about getting Hepatitis or other illness that would trigger my bipolar (depressive phase) and as concerned about putting any vaccine on offer into my body.

Every time I had an 'immune event' (tonsils out, bad case of the flu) I relapsed.

I got a few shots in Thailand as well and had an amazingly good time backpacking in Southeast Asia for nine weeks. I had one major stomach upset in India and contracted a bad virus in Nepal but recovered quickly from both. This therapy is used to treat autoimmune diseases and other medical conditions with IV (intravenous) usage approved by the FDA.

Shark cells oh my. I've had the cells of real, live sharks injected into my tushy… how cool is that? Or maybe it was in the quadriceps muscle of my right, upper thigh? I don't remember clearly. This treatment I had at the height of my illness when I had dropped 25 pounds over the course of a few months without dieting due to body shock from a mugging and sexual assault. At 5 feet 8 1/2 inches tall I weighed a meager 122 pounds.

I was not only sick, I had pretty bad post-traumatic stress disorder symptoms (PTSD).

Live cell therapy is an interesting topic to learn about. An excellent article with information on the history of the therapy, who developed it and how plus why it is used to treat many diseases is *Live Cell Therapy – Questions and Answers*.

Source: Live Cell Therapy - Questions and Answers.
http://www.extendlife.com/livecell.php

165

9. Nutritional Supplements, Tryptophan and Vitamin C

There is an overwhelming amount of information available (books on nutrition, websites, health magazines) on how vitamins and minerals function in the body and how important they are to optimal health. Of course most don't bother to learn about this stuff until they get sick.

When dealing with a chronic illness and the unwanted side effects of prescription medications thinking a natural supplement will cure all that ails you seems like a dream come true. And thinking this way when you have Bipolar I Disorder most likely will lead to crushing disappointment.

At one time I believed the natural amino acid L-Tryptophan would cure me i.e. put an end to the severe depression and mood swings that at times ended in psychosis. No such luck. After I read a book by a psychiatrist who used amino acids to treat depression and regulate moods I got all worked-up about trying this treatment.

Then a bad batch was discovered in Japan that caused a rare yet deadly flu-like illness: Eosinophilia-Myalgia Syndrome (EMS). Shortly thereafter in March, 1990 the FDA banned public sale of L-Tryptophan in the U.S.

It would have been an excellent nutritional supplement for me to try as it functions much like Prozac (increasing levels of serotonin in the brain) without the side effects. You can now only get it by prescription, the FDA does allow that. It became a non-harmful substance when it was something our billionaire pharmaceutical manufacturers could produce and sell.

Or create a chemically-engineered replacement such as Prozac which is then marketed as an approved medical treatment for the same illnesses (depression and anxiety) but only available by a prescription after a costly doctor's visit. What about the cost of required follow-up visits?

Adverse or harmful side effects? People committing suicide?

How backwards is that? And what a shameful disservice to the American public, especially those who suffer from a mood disorder. The below quote is from the *Cognitive Enhancement Research Institute* website:

"The continuing FDA public ban of L-Tryptophan prevents popular access to this most effective serotonin producer. The millions of Americans who for decades safely had relied upon L-Tryptophan to relieve depression, anxiety and PMS, as well as to control pain and induce natural sleep, have been forced elsewhere for solutions."

"Routinely, such solutions are pharmaceutical in nature: people are forced to use either often highly addictive, expensive, and sometimes dangerous drugs like Xanax, Valium, Halcion, Dalmane, Codeine, Anafranil, Prozac, and others, or, simply suffer."

Source: The FDA Ban of L-Tryptophan – Politics, Profits and Prozac

http://ceri.com/trypto.htm

I never did get to try L-Tryptophan for my bipolar illness

but learned much about the pharmaceutical industry and its influence and control over what health care options would be available to me. And about its power and influence over the doctors I would have to go to in order to receive care.

I also learned to stop getting my expectations so high for a natural supplement to be a cure all while continuing my search to get better and feel better.

There are many things you can try that will have an effect on your health and potentially improve your mood states such as sublingual B12, folic acid, B-complex (B6 and B3), vitamin D, amino acids (5-HTP or theanine), etc. Plenty of natural feel-good remedies too such as aromatherapy with essential oils, herbal bath salts, etc.

It is common sense that anyone living with a chronic illness would benefit from a high quality daily multivitamin supplement in addition to eating well, avoiding processed foods and not overindulging in sweets. Healthy living becomes a necessity more than a responsible choice when your mind and body are not in top shape. Unless you want to stay sick and possibly get sicker.

Even better than taking a multivitamin which many don't tolerate well is to buy a Green Food supplement. A couple of capsules taken with water or teaspoons of the nutrient rich green powder added to a smoothie or juice and it is like you consumed ten servings of fruits and vegetables. Without even going shopping or doing any food prep. What bod wouldn't love to be supercharged with that daily?

After researching (and a fair amount of sticker shock) I

decided on the product *Amazing Grass Green Superfood*—150 capsules for only $23. I pop a couple when I think about it, keeping the bottle in the kitchen to remind me to take them along with salmon oil. I encourage my very active and busy teen to take them as well. We eat well but definitely not six or more servings of vegetables and fruits daily. I look at it as cheap health insurance.

It is made out of organic ingredients (wheat grass, spirulina, spinach, chlorella, acai, flax seed powder, apple pectin, etc.), is gluten and GMO free and contains probiotics to keep your gut healthy—no need to buy an acidophilus product separately, saves me cash. You can purchase this product at *Iherb.com*.

Dr. B was focusing on the immune system issues and I had large doses of Vitamin C administered intravenously. This can reduce viral levels in the blood allowing your body to get a break and not be so overwhelmed; help your system get back on fighting ground. You want to stop those offending organisms from holding court in your cells where they have no jurisdiction.

The below is quoted from an abstract of a clinical study on intravenous Vitamin C and its effect on CFS published in the *Medical Science Monitor*:

"Most of these patients had a diagnosis of chronic fatigue syndrome, with the rest being diagnosed as having mononucleosis, fatigue, or EBV infection. Our data provide evidence that high dose intravenous vitamin C therapy has a positive effect on disease duration and reduction of viral antibody levels".

Source: <u>High Dose Vitamin C & Epstein-Barr Viral Infection</u>

http://www.ncbi.nlm.nih.gov/pmc/articles/PMC4015650/

You of course can take Vitamin C orally (by mouth) just in not so high a dose. It is a water soluble vitamin so any excess that is not used by your body will be excreted in your urine or possibly cause loose stools. I take Vitamin C in powder form—2,000 mgs or more daily—whenever I have a cold or the flu. I know being physically sick could trigger a depressive phase and I need to get it under check as quickly as possible.

I have taken *Emergen-C Vitamin C* packets to knock back the start of any viral illness for years. I've also given it to my son whenever he became ill since he was a toddler—trying to avoid having to give him an antibiotic. Each packet contains 1000 mg of Vitamin C plus a small amount of nutrients (to aid in absorption) and antioxidants. It comes in a variety of flavors and you can buy it at Target, Walmart, other in-store pharmacies as well as online.

There are many higher-quality buffered (easy on the stomach) brands of Vitamin C you can purchase in capsule or powdered form. We just have had good luck with *Emergen-C* and it is easy to take. The one drawback is that most of the varieties they offer contain added sugar. On the label it says 'purified fructose'—to your body it is a simple sugar like all others. Buy the lite version or the one that says 'Five Calories' on the label.

Do not try to take large quantities of Vitamin C orally as that can cause serious side effects such as: blood clotting, kidney stones, destruction of red blood cells and even heart-related death.

Source: The Mayo Clinic.com - Vitamin C Safety

http://www.mayoclinic.org/drugs-supplements/vitamin-c/safety/hrb-20060322

One online discount retailer with a large selection—over 30k—of high quality brand name nutritional supplements and other health products (skin care, bath and beauty, grocery items, etc.) is the website mentioned above: *iherb.com*. If you spend $20 or more you get free shipping.

In exploring this path to wellness give yourself credit for being proactive with your health and not just be sitting around waiting for the field of medicine to find a magic potion to cure all that ails you; that may be a while.

10. Salmon Oil

I have saved the best for last i.e. the one nutritional supplement you can easily purchase and take—without a doctor's prescription—that has been proven to affect the brain in ways that may alleviate some of the symptoms of your bipolar illness. Hooray for nutritional science and maverick medical researchers!

The below is quoted from *WebMD.com*:

"Some research suggests that getting more omega-3 fatty acids found in fish oil is linked to greater volume in areas of the brain. In particular, these areas are related to mood and behavior. In one study of 75 patients, one of the benefits of omega-3 fatty acids was decreasing depression in bipolar disorder."

Source: Does Fish Oil Improve Mood with Bipolar Disorder?

http://www.webmd.com/bipolar-disorder/guide/bipolar-diet-foods-to-avoid?page=2#1

I have taken, as mentioned in a previous section, salmon oil at times to the point of almost puking; meaning as much as my stomach would tolerate. It was at one of my 'very sick with bipolar' times and I was desperate for anything to help as I am very intolerant to the majority of psychotropic medications. I was acting erratically (not a big surprise).

It is not necessary to try and overdose on fish oil in hopes of curing your bipolar illness. Not necessary and though relatively harmless will most likely make you feel sick; nauseous, have intestinal gas, loose stools. My new goal is to take 1000 mg of salmon oil a few times a week to keep the levels of those all so important omega-3 fatty acids in a healthy range in my brain. Take that you nasty bipolar-causing genes.

If I had been raised in Japan (same me, same set of genes) eating a traditional Japanese diet consisting of large amounts of fresh fish my mental illness most likely would never have come into being; I'd be normal, not bipolar. Japan has the lowest rate of bipolar illness in the world, insanely low.

The below is quoted from *PsychCentral.com*:

"The people of Japan experience one of the lowest bipolar

disorder rates in the civilized world. Compared to the 4.4 percent lifetime prevalence rate of bipolar disorder in the U.S., in Japan it's just 0.07 percent. That's no typo—that's a crazy large difference."

Source: Can Fish Oil Help Your Brain and Bipolar Disorder?

http://psychcentral.com/blog/archives/2012/09/20/can-fish-oil-help-your-brain-and-bipolar-disorder/

Here is an excellent product I am in the process of starting to take: *Sport Certified Omega-3 Wild Salmon Oil with Vitamin D3.* I want the product that includes the Vitamin D because I was recently told my blood levels were low and advised to start taking a supplement. I hate taking pills so why not do a two-in-one approach.

You can purchase it and other high quality forms of salmon oil online at *VitalChoice.com.*

Whatever supplement you choose, read the label and make sure it contains both EPA and DHA (two types of omega-3 fatty acids), as the two working together is what researchers believe is giving the beneficial effect. A bonus to taking this for your bipolar illness is that it will help your body deal with many other medical conditions; either to prevent them or to treat them. Have a heart condition?

The below quote is from a *WebMD.com* article which lists many medical benefits to taking this supplement:

"People with heart disease are usually advised to take 1 gram (1,000 milligrams) daily of DHA and EPA combined from fish oil.

Source: <u>The Facts on Omega-3 Fatty Acids</u>

http://www.webmd.com/healthy-aging/omega-3-fatty-acids-fact-sheet?page=2

If you have children it would be extremely smart to try and get more fish into their diet and to supplement with salmon oil as well. Why? Besides the health benefits this would give anyone, "The high heritability of bipolar disorder has been well documented through familial incidence, twin, and adoption studies".

Source: <u>Medscape: Bipolar Disorders and Genetics</u>

http://www.medscape.org/viewarticle/489331

None of the above is a panacea but they have helped me and they may help you or a loved one. Important to note is that the descriptions above are of what I have done in addition to traditional therapies when suffering the more serious forms of Bipolar I Disorder and having to be hospitalized as a result. That could have continued beyond my 20s but it didn't.

I do credit being prescribed and taking Synthroid medication as a major turning point in treatment, affecting some of the basic underlying issues that were prompting the severe mood states. And working with Dr. B on treatments that helped my body heal on a physical level, lessen the severe fatigue. Dr. B helped me learn to avoid environmental exposures that were affecting me mentally as well as physically and that has been key to feeling better also.

Not all are so lucky.

In addition to the above I do drink alcohol (red wine, cannot handle hard liquor, stopped drinking beer). I really don't care what the 'bring back prohibition' types think. Moderate alcohol consumption has helped me much in living through and with this illness for many years. It has helped with moods, chronic pain and simply enjoying time with others.

If I was an alcoholic who could not stop drinking if needed it would be another story but I am not. I actually recently decreased my daily intake almost in half, something an addict would not be able to do. I didn't drink during pregnancy or during many other times in my life for extended periods. I choose to imbibe and find it health-promoting like millions of casual and regular drinkers the world over.

If you have to take heavy doses of medication to control your mood swings, or any psychotropic medication on a regular basis, then of course you will have to abstain from alcohol. Drinking alcohol may lessen the effectiveness of your medication, cause an adverse reaction or prompt a biological switch into depression or mania. Not to mention the added stress to your already overtaxed liver.

CHAPTER 16

Learning to Separate Yourself From Illness

T his is a tough one. Really tough and nearly impossible to accomplish when in an active illness state i.e. severe depression or mania. During these times when the railroad tracks have been obliterated, are nowhere to be seen and that derailed train of a brain is a blur in the distance survival is the focus.

You are busy trying to survive the black, bottomless pit of depression without attempting suicide or in a hospital ward after a hypomanic phase progressed to the psychosis of mania. In a psych ward hoping to be released pronto.

"Little one are you still there?"

I spent much of my early 20s not only trying to be well but surviving these extreme states while living life similar to any other bright, Generation X young American at the time. I wanted to have some fun, enjoy time with friends, finish college, make money, have relationships and love in my life. I wanted the diagnosis Manic Depression and all it entailed to go away and never return.

That of course never happened and never will. But what I did eventually learn was how to separate myself a bit from the self that lived through those horrific illness states. To not identify completely with the bipolar illness but to define myself as a person like any other person.

To define myself as someone with intelligence and potential, someone with flaws, positive and negative personality traits; a person with goals and dreams like any other human being has. I learned to put the illness in its place and tell it to leave me the heck alone, is another way to put it. It was a part of me but not the whole of me. I had choices and opportunities like anyone else did.

What I chose to do would determine a large part of who I was and what I accomplished. The illness made life extremely difficult at times but it was not the all of everything I did and of who I was.

It is paradoxical to think of intentionally identifying a part of you as not a part of you. Is that even possible? As well, isn't a primary goal of therapy for someone who has experienced psychosis the reintegration of self?

When the recesses of a mind have been splintered apart involuntarily the first call of action is to patch them back up again, right? You need to alter those brain chemicals in reverse, so to speak. Change them back from being run away cerebral molecules wreaking havoc on anything in their path to sedate, functioning parts of the cell membranes.

You have to first get those train wheel bearings repacked, greased up and rolling again. Now that the crisis has passed and there is some workable machinery with you once again the conductor of your life's journey, then what? What would you like to do now?

This is when you can process that separation of self.

Was it you that created the psychotic episode or severe clinical depression (and most likely involuntary psychiatric hospital stay) you just survived? Or was the psychotic break or major depressive episode caused by an inherited genetic code contained within your body and brain cells that you had little to no control over?

Give yourself credit for surviving then start to rebuild that inner confidence in yourself. You are not the illness. Your illness is simply a part of your life that you have to deal with as best as possible. You are a survivor and a valuable human being. There are people who care and treatment options available to you whenever you are in need of them.

Now think about what you want to do next. Where would you like to be traveling to on that luxury locomotive in first class with the grand, picture glass window framing the gorgeous view outside? What would you like to accomplish now in your life, in the remaining years you have on this planet?

CHAPTER 17

Social Life & Relationships

It was emotionally painful to not have much of a social life when younger. As I got older I learned to enjoy time by myself more and to not stress over what my current friend count is, needing to find a life partner or whether I am getting to do this or that; it's a huge waste of time and energy. I've done many fun things the past two decades and had many enjoyable times with others including travelling to places and countries I never knew I would get to see.

That is enough.

Being alive and not feeling awful, is enough. Surviving Bipolar I Disorder and all that has entailed for over 30 years, that is enough. Still single yet having connecting on many levels with other decent, fun-loving folks throughout my life including a romantic relationship or two, is enough. Having the privilege of parenting a beautiful human being—my son now 18 years old—as a working, single mother; that is more than enough.

I've cooked many tasty meals (plus a few desserts) and shared with family and friends. Photographed people, children and animals all over Latin America and had my photos published along with travel articles I'd written online and in print—small rags, not National Geographic or the New York Times but still. I've created and then sold a small, online, niche website business; written eBooks.

I've swum and snorkeled (one of my favorite hobbies) in oceans on four continents: Asia, North America, South America and Europe. On some occasions the time spent floating in crystal clear, shimmering cobalt blue waters included swarms of sea lions frolicking alongside, blowing bubbles in my face mask: "Hello, I see you, come play with me!"

At other times I swam, diving below the surface over and over again to catch glimpses of the green sea turtle floating nearby that I was joyfully, seamlessly stalking.

When my then 6 year old son and I moved to Mazatlán, Mexico in 2003 we landed at an old run down yet still appealing funky hotel with a very colorful and glamorous past: Hotel Belmar. It was rumored the little alcove at the back of the large, chipped tile, open-air courtyard in front of our small studio apartment was once a writing den of Ernest "Papa" Hemingway—one of the most cherished, respected and emulated American writers of all time.

The loss of this American war hero and formidable intellectual to suicide was partly attributed to his bipolar illness. The below is quoted from a Hemingway biography on *IMDb.com*:

"He was diagnosed with bipolar disorder and insomnia in

his later years. His mental condition was exacerbated by chronic alcoholism, diabetes and liver failure. After an unsuccessful treatment with electroconvulsive therapy, he suffered severe amnesia and his physical condition worsened. The memory loss obstructed his writing and everyday life. He committed suicide in 1961."

Source: Ernest Hemingway Biography

http://www.imdb.com/name/nm0002133/bio

The hotel was located on the malecón (paved promenade) and across the street from the enticing Pacific Ocean with its enchanting swaths of sandy beach. We rode bikes along the waterfront and spent many an afternoon at fancy-pants hotels; with Mom (me) lounging poolside soaking up some therapeutic sunshine while keeping a close eye on the kid who swam and ran himself ragged.

While all this excitement and living life to its fullest was in progress I was careful primarily with two things: the amount of time I spent socializing and going out at night. I simply have to conserve energy and focus on the basic activities of daily living most days, or can push myself over an edge, start to nudge the train off its tracks. Work (when I had a job), school and an occasional night at the bar dancing and playing the pick-up game was tops.

No more off the cuff trips to San Francisco, I told myself. And listen up you too brain.

One time on a job working at an environmental PAC (Political Action Committee) my co-worker and I were in the office together alone and chit chatting the boredom away as we did our work tasks. She was a great gal, brilliant, kind-of crazy like me (though no medical records to prove it, I do have those) and a nice friend at the time.

The conversation started to get a little goofy and we started cracking up. Then I realized as I was laughing that I was starting to not be able to stop laughing. My laughter was elevating and beginning to feel uncomfortable like it was taking on a life of its own, becoming uncontrollable. Uh oh. Relax. Time to chill. No desire to enter Crazyland today thank you very much.

Put on those brakes and keep that train on course.

Limiting social time and becoming much more selective in who I spent the little time I did socialize with helped in becoming stable and maintaining stability, especially when I had a young child to care for. I was (still am) also very aware of my vulnerability as someone with a mental illness and to be careful whom I shared that information with.

I refused to live in silence or fear (still do, hence this book), but you have no choice but to be careful and protect yourself and protect your children. One relationship with a great guy who was a wonderful substitute Dad to my son while we dated was extra special to me since he knew of my history but focused on knowing me as me; and not get freaked out about some medical terminology that has been put in medical records.

That wasn't always the case with attempts at dating or with friendships. You just have to take the ups and downs as they come and keep trying.

When I started travel writing and networking with others online it was a lot of fun as the focus was on work, talent and skills; all of which I had. I fit in well and had the right skill set. The right skills plus loads of passion: I loved traveling, loved living abroad, loved taking photographs and was loving learning how to write and blog about my experiences.

I got travel writing gigs off and on but my main focus was still on parenting my young son and on staying well. I fit in part-time work and freelance assignments as I could, then later branched off on my own. One of those gigs was working for a publishing company in London fact-checking a guidebook to Argentina where we were living at the time. Crappy pay for an overabundance of tedious work but I was thrilled to get the contract. I wanted some extra cash to pay for online courses to add to my son's homeschooling we were doing while living abroad.

A gal from England in the travel writer's group befriended me and we agreed to swap work leads when we could. We never met in person and only chatted a little online. She shared a bit about her divorce, her daughter who was a talented musician and I about living abroad as a single gal with my young son. After the project was complete and I had made some nice contacts with editors at the company I offered to put in a word for her.

Long story short, I helped her get one of the crappy gigs and a short time later mentioned I was bipolar in a communication. That was the end of that, never another written word to me. Not a big deal as was just a casual work connection but illustrates how others react at times after hearing that word and 'you' associated with it. No matter what you accomplish or what kind of person you are.

And I have had many similar experiences over the years.

Unfortunately, the actions of a few can affect the perceptions of the greater whole. Most who were unsupportive or outright hostile had negative experiences with persons who had been labeled with a mental illness and grouped all sufferers together in the same negative light. Or were simply ignorant, mean spirited or both.

Many of those who had known me previously were supportive and caring. Good-hearted souls who knew me as me, not as a psychiatric category. And most twenty-somethings as well as older adults are naturally more focused on working, living their life and having a good time than someone else's problems. A few friends went out of their way trying to be helpful in those early years when I was first diagnosed and I will always be grateful.

I could have passed on the recommendations to read *I Never Promised You a Rose Garden* by a couple of those same friends. It was probably the best they could think of at the time in efforts to be caring and supportive so will let that slide (grin). I try to repay that kindness by being kind-hearted and empathic towards others who are dealing with difficult life stressors.

CHAPTER 18
Care, Concern & Love

Like any illness, persons diagnosed as bipolar deserve care, concern, support and non-abusive treatment options. They may be a pain in the rear end and you may especially want to avoid them if they are Bipolar I and pissed off at you but they—we—are still human beings. We share this planet and are connected to each other on some level whether we like it or not.

In addition, most sufferers did not ask to become ill or do anything knowingly and willingly to cause their illness. And most hate the effect the illness has on themselves, their loved ones and their inability to be high functioning members of society. Like I did and still do. What young person who wants to be out living life, doing great things plus having a little fun at times would not get depressed over feeling tired and ready to pass out around 4 p.m.?

And more depressed when caring, competent physicians could not help? Many would become suicidal under these circumstances, sick of being sick and of having their life force captured by forces outside the realm of their control. Sick of the effort to get well, then feeling better and becoming hopeful only to then downslide into helpless oblivion for no reason.

Like I did.

And many, like I have, would try to fight the illness from various angles when traditional treatment options—i.e. psychotropic medication—were not working. Such as delving into family and relationship issues, trying vitamin and mineral supplements, finding new hobbies, adopting a pet... anything to help. I've done all that and more.

How about leave the country? How about just live your life and forget the whole thing; when you can.

Out of desperation I spent welfare money one time to have a phone consult with a famous psychic. I'd seen her on television many times. They said it cost $400 because she could not afford a car. Wow, what a job. Work for a month and then be driving around town in a Mercedes. It was a few days before I moved into the new living situation then soon after was hospitalized. Her psychic powers predicted none of it. I wanted a refund.

I spent many hours learning how to read Tarot cards. I tried various ways of practicing meditation, tried to understand the basic spiritual concepts of Buddhism. I loved at the time (have since grown out of it) hippy dippy New Age 'out of the box' type of thinking but it doesn't treat serious forms of mental illness, unfortunately. It can offer ways of coping and be a fun pastime or hobby but the illness once obtained remains. You are partners for life.

And the gay issue—that kept on for years and there were more offensive, intending to be mean jabs such as: "They have observed pigs doing it". I had become a suspected lesbian. Oh my, who stamped that on my forehead? Not I. Didn't do wonders for attempts at dating, but did give me some things to try and entertain Sexy 2 with during our weekly sessions since my life was pretty boring at the time.

I had my leg felt up on a few occasions in attempts to entice some action; no thank you. Left a job after being sexually harassed by an older (ick) lesbo.

The concept wasn't a big deal and I wasn't homophobic but it definitely bothered me. I wasted a lot of time reading erotica and 'coming out' stories but ended up back to what I already knew. Yes some of it was a turn on but it wasn't my wiring or my thing. Maybe I was a little confused, inexperienced but is that such a bad thing? A little confusion and needing lessons can lead to some hot exploration.

I was (still am) a bit odd in the social sense but it didn't have to do with some deep, hidden attraction to women; no secret childhood crushes except to older men. I'm the oversensitive type plus a bit shy and immature in some ways, not to mention being forced to spend quite a bit of my personal time simply dealing with illness.

And who would want me anyways other than for a nice, casual good time? I did have a few of those, though am not into being used.

I had a mental illness and didn't really have a good grasp on the situation, it wasn't being controlled, many things were contributing to it and I had little stability to count on with regards to myself. A relationship requires a sharing of one's self and an underlying respect for each other. Face it, most people will fear someone they find out has dealt with mental illness not respect them.

That is the true crux of the suffering this illness doles out: forced instability. You get a bit better then are slammed with a new episode of depression. Or get a bit better then realize I am starting to wind up. I am laughing a little too hard, thinking a little too fast and that hypomanic state I am entering into could lead to full-on mania and hospitalization. Toss that supplement/drug/therapy book into the trash. Time to eat another bowl of popcorn as that is about all I will be able to afford today on welfare assistance.

Job, life, love... when you are a young twenty-something there is that little nagging question of what to do with your life. Why have you been put on this planet and are you living up to your potential or just screwing off. So you are bipolar. So what.

Answering those questions when you have the background static of mood ups and downs—the ups making you feel capable of doing anything and coming out of the downs feeling like you are a pathetic and complete failure for not succeeding—is not an easy task. But they should be asked and need to be asked. You have to still think of the future, not let the illness control your entire life, all moments of your life. Especially when the illness hits at a young age.

And remind yourself off and on that everyone is screwed up a bit, not just you.

Then things level out and basic life resumes. That normal,

functioning self is back cruising around yet with another notch on the 'illness taking its toll' pole. You have a few good months, good years, enjoy life. Until a new episode comes to the forefront and your psyche once again kicks into gear with its laser sharp critical assessments flooding the consciousness over and over again.

What is your potential anyways, it asks? Is it an underused high IQ shrouded in mental illness. Or like anyone else, are you just not working hard enough, trying hard enough, setting goals and sticking with them until they are met. Needing to do what anyone else who accomplishes anything in life needs to do.

And didn't a lot of famous, brilliant folks suffer the same, if not worse, thing? The internal dialogue continues without much restraint. Am I being grandiose to assume I am capable of achieving higher levels of functioning or am I truly a part of a select group of human beings who have the genetic code that gives greatness its spark, creativity its undercurrent that lies await until the inevitable flood of brilliance?

And if I'm so great and so smart... why am I so poor and alone? That was always a tough one. When I improved in my late 20s by successfully treating underlying issues that were causing the more extreme moods and mood swings much of that obsessive thinking and ruminating ended. I had also found something that worked for the chronic pain condition which was adding to the depressive states and fatigue—the OTC pain reliever Aleve.

I started to become too busy with life to bother, not stuck anymore in a mental prison where all I really had for company were my thoughts. And thankfully I matured some. I gave birth to my son at age 31 and then had little time to daydream or self-criticize. The focus was on working, raising him as a single parent and keeping myself healthy. The bipolar stayed in the background, Crazyland was kept at bay yet I knew it was there. And was just hoping it would stay put and not cause me any problems or need for treatment.

As you move through life living with this illness and affecting illnesses like CFS, hypothyroidism, multiple sclerosis, arthritis or anything else someone can suffer from, things change even if you don't. Medical doctors gather to discuss new research and come up with new diagnostic categories and standards of treatment. Drug companies rush to meet the demands of mood-altering drugs and potential cures of mental illness.

Or at least perceived cures in lieu of marketing more product.

CHAPTER 19

We Will Skip the Torture

As time goes on and new medical discoveries are made the dynamics of mental illness becomes more understood or can be altered to fit the mood of the day. I think two things make a DSM category: medical research as well as current trends in thinking. And trends change such as the shift in thought post 1980 from maladaptation as a result of character weakness and lack of discipline to illness from a biologically-induced disease process; if I am understanding correctly.

Changes in treatment protocols may follow like the move away from behavior modification and punishment to attempts at identifying underlying biochemical processes and medications which will lessen their adverse effects. The patient may have extreme mood states or personality issues but how much of that is the result of—or exacerbated by—their brain chemistry? Their particular genetic profile and the expression it has taken due to outside forces, not free will.

Who or what is controlling that Crazyland wallpaper? That is more of the question than how self-disciplined a person is.

That's my creative take on it. A more professional inside scoop synopsis is given by psychologist Judith Schlesinger in her critically acclaimed book *The Insanity Hoax: Exposing the Myth of the Mad Genius* published in January, 2012.

"Officially, the DSM does not presume to describe illness, yet terminology like 'symptom', 'remission', and 'clinical' gives it a distinctly medical whiff and weight. Moreover, it presents its categories as if they were just as real as a heart attack."

"But heart attacks don't require negotiation to exist. In contrast, mental disorders are hammered out by backstage argument full of intra-guild squabbling and self-interested trading (I'll support your new disorder if you'll vote for mine), and—all too often—corruption. At one recent point, every expert working on the depression category had financial ties to the pharmaceutical industry."

Source: The Insanity Hoax: Exposing the Myth of the Mad Genius

http://www.theinsanityhoax.com/

Psych docs tell their story of how and why the DSM came into being from its inception in 1952 to current times including information on how mental illnesses are classified on the *American Psychiatric Association* website: History of the DSM.

http://www.psychiatry.org/psychiatrists/practice/dsm/history

Beyond the debate over psychiatric diagnostic categories, let's hope government officials never play a major role in how we define and treat mental illness for many reasons though they usually get their two cents in anyways. Why keep those types of people in power to the wayside of the discussion? Think like this.

Was Frances Farmer gang raped by soldiers in the 1940s in the back ward of a mental hospital at the approval of licensed (by the state) medical personnel because of an assumed affiliation to a belief in Communism since she happened to win a trip to the Soviet Union in college for a scholastic achievement?

Was that the real reason she was held captive to those white walls for an approximate five years and repeatedly subjected to various forms of torture? Was it a form of political persecution more than treatment of a mental illness?

We have come a long way and need to keep playing it forward.

Or how about her religious beliefs? She was a self-professed agnostic (not an atheist or a Christian) and wrote an essay in high school (another award winner) titled, "God Dies". What would some overzealous folks even today in 2015 think of that and possibly consider it cause to target the teen?

In September, 1997 a right-wing, evangelical Christian group from the U.S. traveled to Kathmandu, Nepal to hold a prayer marathon in the Himalaya mountain range. A range famous for climbing expeditions on Mount Everest—the highest mountain in the world. During their time seeking God's guidance and evidence of some form of divine intervention Mother Teresa happened to pass away. She was

87 years old and being cared for at the Missionaries of Charity headquarters in Kolkata, India.

The female leader of the evangelical group claimed partial credit for her passing. She rejoiced in the death of this most cherished saint of a woman who was awarded the Nobel Peace Prize in 1979 for her service to the poor. Mother Teresa's coincidental time of passing from this earth during their stay on the mountain was looked at by these Christian radicals as a sign from God; a sign of the power of their prayer.

Are these people mentally ill? Genetically pre-programmed to become evil? Let's keep the religious fanatics out of the discussion too, they have their churches and freedoms, others should as well.

Lastly, maybe a bit of concern should be directed at what is going on at the institutions training our mental health care providers. Professors at UCSF who taught and awarded Doctorate degrees to the 'Trio Three PhDs' has to be looked at as a primary cause that created the group think harassment I was subjected to.

What about other universities and their effect on treatment of those diagnosed with mental illness? What are these programs teaching?

There is an Oxford University professor who is advocating for altering the personality of fetuses in utero. Yes, that is correct. The 'how' this would be done is beyond absurd (this guy surely needs a shrink) but what is far worse is the fact not only that he thinks it can be done but that it SHOULD be done. Something about a 'moral obligation'. Please tell me that makes you cringe too.

Another mad scientist (this one in the states) believes he has found God by creating a torture machine. Wow, and don't sign me up. What happened to the premise 'God is love'? Or maybe (more of the understanding I have come to from learning about different religions) simply a compilation of energy—a spirit force. An energy potential within all of us, contained within our collective DNA blueprint.

We all have the capacity to be godlike. To be decent human beings who care about others. If that is more of what the truth is, then maybe God is being destroyed by those who think they are god. By those who are egotistical and arrogant enough to think—believe—they are doing God's work.

From bad blood, possession by evil spirits, inadequate mothering to genetic vulnerability and lack of or overproducing brain chemicals; the causes and treatments of diagnosable mental illnesses change over time. Where will it go next in regards to bipolar illness?

In giving thought to that question let's skip the 'altering fetuses in utero' proposition and torture as treatment too. We here in the U.S. and around the world can do better than that.

We can all work towards continuing the trend away from punishment to an ongoing search for effective medical treatments. A search each and every one of us can participate in. We can all walk alongside the dedicated, caring doctors, nurses, psychologists, medical researchers and mental health advocates who lead the way. We can work together and help each other.

None of us is separate from the whole of human existence and no one is alone.

One of the most touching experiences of my pre-illness teenage years was in being asked to participate in a 'spiritual search' boot camp of sorts. I already mentioned I was raised in a Catholic family and attended Catholic schools, this was something someone in that community came up with for a rite of passage for teenagers.

I thought all it entailed was going on a camping trip and participating in a few group talks about issues and decision-making coming to the forefront such as sex, marriage, learning more of the history and traditions of the church, etc. Birth control and the prevention of unwanted pregnancies would have been a pertinent topic to discuss for this age group but was left off the agenda.

It was in a beautiful location and all participants had a good time. I recall something about underwear gone missing at night then found up in a tree outside the next morning upsetting those in charge a bit but the main goals were met notwithstanding a few antics.

What I didn't expect was to receive a packet of letters at the end of the weekend, to be opened in private. The packet contained a mix of writings from a variety of folks who knew me in some form or the other and had stayed up all night holding a prayer vigil for the attendees. Talk about touching. I was impressed they had stayed up all night much less taken the time to write kind notes for everyone.

That type of search and sharing we all can do at any time during our lives and for anyone. We can search spiritually inside ourselves and share what we learn with others if we so choose. We can attend church services and be devoted to a particular religious doctrine and its dogma. We can learn about Eastern Mysticism or study the ancient dark arts.

Or we can simply be good people. The type of persons who have care and concern about the well-being of others in addition to our selves—like so many in the mental health field who not only assist persons diagnosed with mental illness but have fought for better treatment of and treatment options for all sufferers for decades.

CHAPTER 20

Living Life & Moving On

W hen you write a personal memoir and come to the end you reach the present. At this time (year 2015) my son and I live in the U.S. after around nine years traveling and living abroad: Spain, Canada, Mexico, Guatemala, Nicaragua, Costa Rica, Panama, Ecuador, Argentina, Bolivia and Peru.

My son is a bright, healthy, bilingual and biliterate teen who loves to snowboard and wants to be a chef. I do a mix of writing, editing, blogging and trying to figure out new ways to make money on a part-time work schedule. If you need a talented freelancer for a project (large or small) check out my portfolio and shoot me an email: Online Portfolio.

http://www.mollymchugh.com/molly-mchugh-online-portfoliocv/

How about help writing, designing and publishing an e-book?

Before moving abroad, after around 18 years of surviving the illness and episodes, I successfully applied for social security disability (SSDI). Due to a high functioning period with well-paid work in the tech field while raising my son as a single mother the amount awarded was sufficient to allow me to start a new life outside of the U.S. A life where I could afford a decent level of living, have some fun and expose my child to other cultures, languages and ways of living.

It was exhilarating to win the claim but I felt a lot of shame about qualifying for support. I never feel shame about having a mental illness—that is outside my realm of control and is just a tough break in a sense, being dealt a bad hand. But it was humiliating to not be self-supporting. Working and living in the world successfully is something competent, healthy adults are supposed to have a handle on.

If you don't, you're a loser.

When meeting new people it was embarrassing to say I was receiving a pension when people wanted to know what work I did. It would have been much easier to lie and claim to be a trust fund baby or techie turned millionaire yet I didn't. Most were just curious fellow expats (American, Canadian, European) and not rude enough to press for details but if someone did, I simply said I "had a mix of health issues"—which is the truth.

The locals never asked. I was American, therefore automatically assumed to be rich.

I did finally get back to some part-time, professional work (travel writing, blogging and e-books) and that did help my sense of self-worth much. It helped me feel better about myself and affirmed that I wasn't being lazy or taking advantage of the system. I was doing the best I could with what I had to work with and was a responsible, loving mother. If I could not work full time because of serious health issues it was not something I should be beating myself up over.

As a single mother of a young child my days included plenty of work.

I was stable with the bipolar for long periods of time after my 20s but still had other health issues. And don't forget... stable for a person diagnosed with Bipolar I Disorder means in part no major depressive or manic episodes resulting in hospitalization. That doesn't mean I didn't have down times or some high times, as is the norm for a major mood disorder, I did. I just struggled with life like others do and kept myself out of the psych void.

Someone with a less severe version of the illness may suffer much, need treatment and medication but—lucky them—rarely to never see the inside of a psych ward. Have I mentioned the heavy, steel-reinforced doors (usually grey), steel locks and metal mesh screened windows yet? Seriously, it is not an experience you would want to have but if so inclined can go ahead and wish it on your worst enemy. Some sick people live free and harm others much with their victim the one who ends up in a locked ward.

I also mention a sexual assault and of being mugged (both in my 20s) in the text above, though did not elaborate on either. This book was not meant to be a crime saga or a pity party is one reason. The other reason is that weaving in those issues would have clouded the description of my experiences living and receiving treatment for the bipolar; a biochemically-induced mood disorder. That is what I wanted to focus on, not personal dramas.

In addition, if I had tried to go that route this book would never have been written. Having to process and think of then write about the sexual assault (the offender was not punished but it did not go unreported and that is significant) was what prevented me from finishing the project years ago. It was too much to have to mentally rehash, to try and recall dates this or that happened, etc.

The assault was during a medical exam. I blacked out during the incident and for months after (no alcohol involved) yet had no idea why at the time. Then years later during a sexual relationship it resurfaced and again had blackouts. I was stimulated and brought to orgasm during the assault.

It added a lot of confusion to my treatment (I believe it was Sexy 2 at the time or soon after I ended that care), a lot of confusion to me as well as to what the hell was my problem. Why was I crying for no reason? Why when I opened my mouth would no words come out? It took over a year to recall what I could remember and then deal with it.

The mugging was a year or so later. It was not overly-traumatic, the offender was caught and charged. He had just been released from a heroin detox facility I was told. Twisting of my neck and back caused injury that didn't respond well to treatment. During the assault I was pulled down a set of stairs and the purse I had strapped around my neck was torn off. Then I tried to run—limp—after the guy.

The twisting created a chronic pain condition called fibromyalgia.

Those things were being dealt with in the background

when the bipolar would take center stage, so you can understand why I had the extent of treatments I did and visits to a bunch of docs. The majority of treatments I received were thankfully covered under the state Crime Victims Compensation fund.

I also left out other 'nurture' type of stuff (we have been focusing on the nature aspects) such as family issues, childhood traumas. I had repeated nightmares as a child of someone entering the home, coming up the stairs into my room and onto my bed, then jumping on the bed over my body... was in terror, paralyzed, could not move; woke up screaming. Sometimes then walked down the hall and climbed in bed with my parents, other times cried myself back to sleep.

Walked and talked in my sleep a few times. Sucked my thumb at night and wet my bed way past typical timeframes. Youngest of five children, two year older brother got me to climb a tree right into a bee's nest one time (yes, much scrambling, screaming and running ensued plus a sting or two).

My beloved pet gerbil "Herbie the Love Bug" passed away when I was 16 and I was devastated. I may have been two weeks shy of kindergarten when I learned to tie my shoes properly but really can't remember and they didn't penalize kids for such things back then.

In 8th grade my teacher kept me in the classroom alone for a few minutes before recess to talk. Exasperated with my over-exuberance he told me I was "acting like a chicken with its head cut off". I later learned he soon after left the school to teach at an all-boys high school. I choose to believe there is no correlation between the two events.

When I was around 12 years old I put God to the test. I walked by myself on a weekday morning (must have been a school vacation or summer) to our local church and sat in a pew. Just sat, thought, looked around; only one or two other parishioners there, no priest. And waited. Didn't feel much. It felt comforting to be in the building which was lovely but I was looking for something more.

Wondered if God and church were a sham and why the starlings that used to wake me up in the mornings with their loud chitter chatter outside my bedroom window had all but gone away. "I'm going to shoot those crows," my Dad used to say.

And then I'd spend weeks, months wondering if it was ok, ok to shoot the crows. They were eating all the starling eggs but could we shoot them, was that ok? Could never decide. There's a lot of crap and psychological drama in everyone's past.

When I got out of what was to be my last major hospitalization (age 26 or so) I was going to write this book but could never get through the first few sentences until years later. I wanted to participate in life with some value, contribute something positive out of the hell I had endured like many others before me. I think there should be a specific literary genre for 'Mental Illness Memoirs'.

Maybe this book should have been granted the title: "Psych Patient".

Many of those books written by those courageous authors were the only thing that helped me survive some of the bad times, times when no one else and nothing medically was helping. Help that was during the downswing of the experience. At the high-end was hypomania or mania and I usually wasn't in the mellow 'read a book' mood.

I wanted to list them here but have forgotten the titles of most of them so it wouldn't be fair to list only the few I could pull up now via an Internet search. There wasn't Amazon back then and some I found and read in other countries. I will say one of my favorites, since at the time I fancied myself an aspiring journalist after finishing college with a B.A. in Communications was *The Beast: A Journey Through Depression* by Tracy Thompson, published in 1996.

I related a lot to what this former Washington Post investigative reporter went through and her account of her experiences with depression and treatments for depression; including her experience of being hospitalized and then having a therapist abandon her as she was deemed unworthy of care after that, somehow weak to succumb to such a horrible fate.

She was not bipolar but suffered much.

Books on bipolar were uncommon back then (personal accounts) but now in the year 2015 almost passé. There are a lot of them, many I now want to read after having done an Internet search. The last book on mental illness I read in 2001 before my son and I moved abroad. It was *An Unquiet Mind: A Memoir of Moods and Madness* by Kay Redfield Jamison; loved it. She was giving a talk in Seattle at the time near where we lived and I wanted to go but couldn't wing it.

Like Jamison I have tried to give a firsthand account of what it is like to live with bipolar illness; a descriptive lens into the process as a whole. A kaleidoscope perspective of sorts of living with and through the myriad of symptoms for years on end. And I did not shy away from sharing some of the outer effects such as discrimination sufferers may face, how others may perceive you.

I hope this book has helped you to understand some of what a person who has bipolar illness may experience and some things that might help them improve their health. Things that may lessen the severity of the disease and the suffering it causes, especially if they have been diagnosed with Bipolar I Disorder.

Or if you are one of those people given you some comfort, made you feel not so alone or without hope and possibly a giggle or two. Come on, '...invent a new form of zipper'? That's funny!

As well I hope an element of celebration has shone through in this sharing. A celebration of and tribute to all who have fought to improve the lives of the unfortunate 5.7 million Americans (2.6% of the U.S. population 18 years or older) who are diagnosed with bipolar disorder in any given year.

Source: Brain & Behavior Research Foundation.

https://bbrfoundation.org/frequently-asked-questions-about-bipolar-disorder

I wish you the best on your journey, Molly

P.S. You can write a review of this book on Amazon.

Website: www.mollymchugh.com

Facebook: www.facebook.com/ bipolar1survivor

Bipolar 1 Survivor blog: www.bipolar1survivor.com

Made in the USA
Las Vegas, NV
07 September 2021